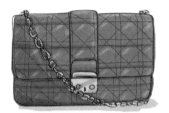

NATHALIE PEIGNEY

SOPHIE *the* PARISIAN

STYLE TIPS FROM A
TRUE PARISIAN WOMAN

With illustrations by
Alessandra Ceriani

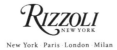

RIZZOLI
NEW YORK

New York · Paris · London · Milan

To my mother,
so pleased to be Parisian!

WHAT IS
A PARISIAN?

*A charming woman, often chic but complex
and paradoxical. To be more specific: someone who
can be charming without an ultra-bright smile,
and chic in blue jeans.*

The Parisian has an elusive personality that's hard to pin down. At first, she comes off as distant and a little cold. But fairly quickly you realize she's refined but nice. She's saucy, with a stinging sense of humor. She likes to surprise you. She'll open up when you least expect it, then suddenly pull back into her shell, and finally go back to being her charming self again.

Everybody talks about Parisian charm. Perhaps part of our charm stems from being mysterious. We're like hidden, genetically programmed behavior codes that only other Parisians know how to read and use. You hear a lot about French attitude or typical Parisian behavior. Well, I guess it's true. We have typical ways of acting with our friends, our men, our kids, and strangers. We know what we want and how to get it, but we won't reveal too much of our strategy behind this natural and innocent-looking appearance.

There's the native Parisian, born and bred in Paris, and then there's the "Parisian by adoption." As it turns out, it can be hard to tell them apart. Fortunately, you don't have to be born Parisian to become Parisian. According to Karl Lagerfeld, "you don't even have to be French to be Parisian"—provided, however, that you have a good friend like me, a benevolent godmother who takes you under her wing and reveals all the tricks of the trade. And, of course, provided you have the proper guide from which to extract essential pearls of wisdom as needed. Be careful: becoming Parisian is possible, but remaining Parisian is an art. It takes a lot of work to achieve the supreme result: perfect style that looks natural and spontaneous. One day you'll finally manage, but watch out—there's no letting up. One slip and you're a "has been." Not that I want to be discouraging. Hang in there and follow my advice. Write my tips on Post-its and stick them on the fridge, on your bathroom mirror, and on the dashboard of your car. In no time, "Parisian-ness" will soon become an automatic reflex.

Another part of our appeal is the way we mix our grandmothers' traditions with the latest trends. We dream of traditional dishes with rich sauces but nourish ourselves on steamed *haricots verts* (French beans) with barely a dash of olive oil. We enjoy simple and light *nouvelle cuisine* but also love not-so-light Italian recipes that we happily blend into our own culinary heritage. This is sometimes known as "the French paradox." It is the art of masterfully juggling styles, of nimbly shifting back and forth between apparently contradictory trends. It is an acquired skill.

We're brought up to be careful about the way we speak; language is part of our image and bearing. Yet we don't hesitate to adapt some of the "in" expressions of our teenage children, which are not always refined but are an unavoidable part of urban life. Pop slang one moment, literary discussion the next—it's not always easy to keep up with our conversation, but that's just the way it goes, for the Parisian does not have a moment to spare!

We are said to be elegant. Even if our style is meticulously planned, it must look very natural. Once again, we have our little secrets. There are strict rules for being and staying chic, whether we're getting married, strolling the banks of the Seine, or sipping a cocktail at *Café de Flore,* a legendary sidewalk café in the quaint Saint-Germain-des-Prés district. The same goes for our kids. They must be well bred, well behaved, and impeccably dressed: the small Parisians!

My girlfriends in the States are always telling me how Parisian I am and asking me for advice on shopping and style. I take the compliments with all due modesty. Of course, I know all the right addresses in the French capital for just about everything—from the fanciest chocolate éclair to the best private sales. I'm very proud to share my "finds," but only rarely will I actually divulge my "secret" addresses. A *Parisienne* wouldn't be a *Parisienne* without her little black book of the "right places." After all, whether you're looking for a soup bar, a hat boutique, or a health spa, "in" is "in," "out" is "out."

The Parisian is said to be svelte. But do we ever love our pastries, sausage, and cheese! How do we keep the weight off? Let's say that we are constantly on guard, preferring the philosophy of "preventing and correcting" to that of "repairing and healing."

Last but not least, the Parisian woman would not be what she is without Paris, a city that is sublime but often gray, an exciting place but also a tough one. Paris is a magnificent setting, a stage for the greatest celebrities of our time. Paris is also a demanding place to live. If you are worthy of the *Ville Lumière* (City of Light), you won't be seen dead in baggy sportswear or floppy shoes. Paris is a city where people are expected to outdo themselves. There are strict rules here about what is and isn't done. If one is or aspires to be Parisian, one behaves as expected 24/7, even when traveling. Paris is a harsh mistress, but the Parisian bends to her strict rules and criticism with pride. She is proud of the beauty of the city and its cultural riches. This pride can be sensed in her character.

To keep her face looking naturally youthful even as time marches on, to keep her figure despite a sweet tooth, and to live up to her famous reputation, the Parisian woman must constantly have the right attitude at the right moment. Ready to learn?
I'll be here to help you become an authentic Parisian woman, supported by testimonials by my girlfriends, all strictly Parisian women.

Now it's up to you to choose the first word.

Nathalie Peigney

How to use this book

Sophisticated, curious, eclectic, paradoxical ... how could one possibly sum up the essence of my Parisian friends in just a few adjectives? A multitude of words comes to mind to evoke the Parisian lifestyle, and it's so hard to choose. So I dropped 103 emblematic terms into my hat, and I leave it to you to draw the magic words that will open the gates of Parisian style for you.

You'll find classics like *Attitude, Femininity, Grayness, Luxury, Black, The Place to Be*, and *Ville Lumière* as well as essentials such as *Baguette, Bidet, Bistro, Croque-monsieur, French Kiss, Little Black Dress,* and *Vinaigrette*, all of which depict typical Parisian life. In addition to the words that accompany my professional life in the French capital, there are many others regarding a more private but also fashionable and trendy realm with family and friends, at school, at the market, upon awakening, or during happy hour. Naturally there are terms for mouthwatering foods and others more ... intimate. The wordlist appears in alphabetical order from A to Z, but feel free to jump around and pick items at random or read in whatever order you like, since the idea is to share tidbits of Parisian life and give you tricks and tips for becoming something of a Parisian woman yourself. I hope the words will also intoxicate you with the fragrances, sounds, and colors of the town. Imagine the aroma of croissants fresh out of the oven, sparrows singing in the Place de Dauphine, the colorful richness of the city's outdoor markets, and the joys of Paris window-shopping—all the feelings that shape the personality and sensitivity of the Parisian! My little glossary is intended to be fun, but it is 100% authentic and comes from close observation.

Sometimes the depiction of the Parisian woman in these pages is a deliberate cliché that must not be taken too literally and should be applied with discretion and finesse by anyone seeking to emulate the true Parisian look and attitude. "Less is more" is an insight into Parisian chic that you should keep in mind as you read. Here I pass on my secrets the way I do for my best friends, so please do not disappoint me when applying them!

Here is a simple and easy-to-digest little book to read (and re-read) anywhere, any time: in the metro, between meetings, at bedtime. I'm going to talk to you about fashion, cooking, seduction, and little quirks that make us so charming, and about our children, the way only real Parisians talk.

The pictures in this book portray a twenty-first-century Parisian woman, in various situations of her life: biking on the Place des Vosges, on the way to the office, in her kitchen, on the terrace of a café in her little black dress before going out to dinner, rushing to an appointment, reading on her balcony, out shopping with her best friends or her husband. The focus is on the Parisian herself but also on the streets and squares of Paris —fundamental visual images that translate the vibrancy and vitality of the fascinating *Ville Lumière* in constant motion.

LINKS
To learn more about the topic, go directly to the entries that interest you.

MY TIP
These are to be taken with due caution: a personal note that comes from my experience is not an absolute dictate.

HISTORY
Brief, interesting, and/or entertaining information that you should know to grasp the pure essence of an entry.

THE RECIPE
I added a small, entirely personal ingredient to the traditional recipes, transforming the final result.

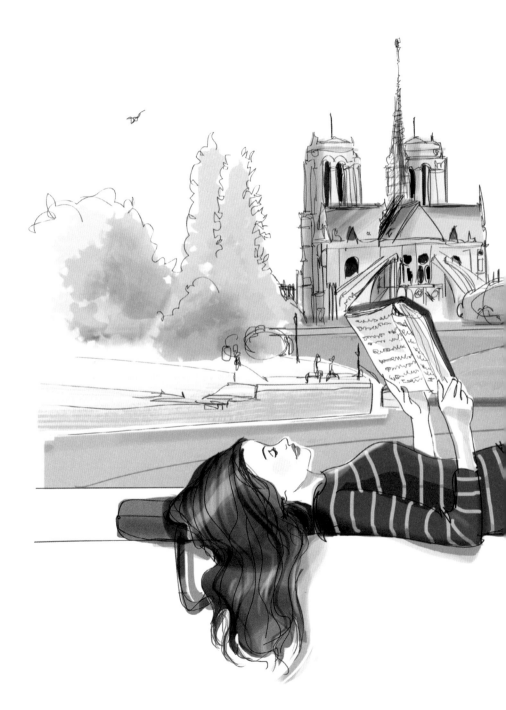

103 THINGS TO KNOW TO BE LIKE HER

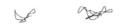

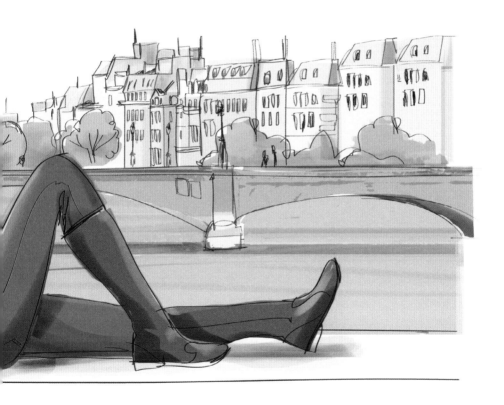

A

Accessories

In Paris, an accessory is not, as the *Merriam Webster* dictionary defines it, "a thing of secondary or lesser importance"—it's a fundamental part of the Parisian woman's look. An outfit without the right belt or scarf or casual chic bag to go with it would be missing something; it would be too bland. Accessories are the "salt and pepper" of style, and that's why they are so important to a woman's wardrobe. If a Parisian needs to pack lightly for a trip, she'll take just three basics—her little black dress, a pair of jeans (the good ones), and a trench coat—but she wouldn't even think of leaving without taking a dozen good accessories to diversify her attire. If you really want to emulate Parisian style, start by learning how we choose accessories!

• Don't coordinate. The Parisian is a free spirit. Composition is a contemporary art that she loves, unlike her grandmother, who went for a "total" look. She would never put a fuchsia *Saint-Laurent* bag with *Roger Vivier* or *Repetto* ballerina shoes just because they're the same pink.

• Mix values and styles. It's more elegant. A designer or luxury accessory like an *Isabel Marant Fauna* belt or *Ileana della Corte* earrings adds class to an inexpensive

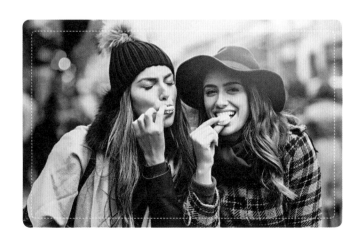

LINKS
• Bag
• Shoes
• Vintage
• Wardrobe

black dress. Or you can take the opposite tack: a minimalist bracelet or an ethnic accessory can be the magic touch to tone down a look that might otherwise be too dressy. I love wearing fun mini *Tabio* socks with my black evening sandals!

• Wear only things you like and/or that look good on you. Who said you have to wear a striped *Dries Van Noten* scarf or *Charlotte Olympia* platform heels to have a drink at *Café de Flore* in Saint-Germain-des-Prés? A Parisian never feels forced to act like anyone else, including movie stars. She keeps an eye on the fashion shows and what's trending but refuses to be a fashion victim.

• Wear a belt every day. Some of the advantages: it makes an androgynous figure more glamorous, shows off your small waist, adds a Parisian signature to your look, or gives your pants some pep by playing with contrast.

• Always have pairs of basic shoes in your closet (flats, black heels, sandals, boots, ballerina shoes, and loafers). Buy only the right size and height for you. Leave the five-inch-heel *Jimmy Choos* in the store if you can't walk gracefully in them.

• Clean, iron, and shine! Keep your accessories in good shape if you want to look chic.

• Don't accept fakes. If you can't afford a genuine luxury bag, get one that's simple but made of nice leather. The true *Parisienne* buys a bag because she's fallen in love with it—not because it's a famous brand. Luxury means quality, not price.

• Use bags like Russian matryoshka dolls (one nesting inside the other) to cover various needs. For example, stick a *Balenciaga* evening clutch inside an *Upla* shoulder bag or in a *Vanessa Bruno* tote bag.

• Avoid "chichi" frilly hats. Sobriety is a sign of elegance. To get an idea of what's stylish, check out the designer hat makers: *Atelier 144, Gilles François, Lanvin, Maison Michel.* Choosing the right hat, whether for a wedding or for everyday wear, is no easy matter. The Parisian just makes it seem easy.

MY TIP
Wear your accessories with as much ease and spontaneity as possible. Try to tie, wrap, fit at the waist, and mix several times before leaving the house, and avoid a "cherry on the top" style that makes you feel uncomfortable. Remember, the *Parisienne* is sure of herself and her style.

- Opt for nice material and fabrics. A leather belt, not a nylon one; a mohair scarf, not viscose. They're nicer to wear, prettier, and not necessarily more expensive.
- Leave anything with flashy designer labels at the back of your closet. Bling is not Parisian.
- Play culture fusion. Wear a boyish *Comptoir des Cotonniers* pea coat with a *Jhin* Japanese-style pocket square.
- Tame the savage beast. Keep your zebra, leopard, or panther on a short leash—in other words, wear animal looks sparingly, just to accent your look from time to time.
- Wear oversize sunglasses. Always have a pair handy that you can whip out as soon as a sunbeam bursts from the Paris sky.

Age

A proper French upbringing encourages little girls (not just little boys) to develop their personalities and to do well at school rather than to waste time admiring themselves in a mirror. This is also essentially the approach at religious schools, where, until recently, the notion of feminine fulfillment did not really exist and where focusing too much on one's physical appearance was considered the height of futility. Thus the Parisian woman learns from a tender age to develop her inner beauty. When she reaches the age of physical seduction, this inner beauty reinforces her charm and the radiance of her face. And when she eventually reaches an age when her figure is no longer her main asset, the true Parisian

MY TIP
The *Parisienne* is attentive to detail (take care of your teeth, hands, and feet before it's too late); she's careful about what she says, how she says it, and her body language; she knows how to show off her best feature, whether it's her figure or the way she looks at you. Last, but not least, the Parisian woman does her best to eat right. Fad diets are out! She knows that proper nutrition is the way to age in good health.

LINKS
- Class
- Grandma
- Hair
- Madeleine

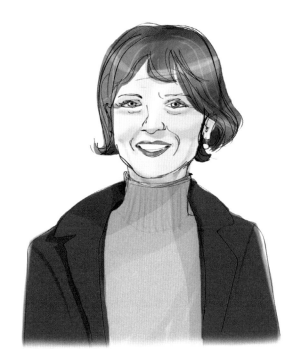

is not disheartened, for she has other cards to play: her charisma and her interior charm. She has prepared herself intellectually to face the aging process. She is curious and inherently interested in all kinds of cultural and social events. She has attended, has heard of, or is dying to find out about every imaginable show or exhibition in the city. There is no event about which she does not have a strong personal opinion that she is happy to express at great length to her friends.

The Parisian also knows that after age fifty, there are a few things she will have to give up. She knows the limits of her body and face. She is perfectly aware that, to age gracefully, the worst thing she can do is to dress like a teenager and to rely on physical charms indefinitely. Trying to make time stand still is a lost cause and being pessimistic about growing older is self-defeating. It's cooler to accept your age and throw your energy into developing your charm. Opening your mind, satisfying your curiosity, quenching your thirst for life, and staying fit are the only ways to beat age! Looking at people more gently and taking the time to truly understand them gives your face a charming softness it didn't have at age twenty-five. Gray hair? Leave the "salt and pepper" look to men. In Paris, you either hide gray hair entirely or show it off if the "I'm proud of my age" look becomes you.

Things the older Parisian woman has going for her: she keeps weight off by watching what she eats and walking a lot; her hair is well cared for; she uses plastic surgery sparingly (100% wrinkle-free would be a big mistake, since smile lines, for example, make you look more beautiful, not less); she's got class (nobody over fifty wants to dress girlishly anymore—who wants to be mocked as an "over-the-hill Lolita"?); she wears 1½-inch heels to elongate her figure and wears mostly soft or neutral colors; she has spent her life taking almost compulsive care of her skin; she applies makeup for a simple yet feminine look.

Aperitif

In Paris, the aperitif is a sacred rite; less demanding and more expeditious than a dinner, it allows the Parisian woman to see her friends or meet a potential boyfriend without staying out too late. And the capital is bustling with good places for a romantic or friendly drink.

Here the question is not the program of Parisian nights, which offer all kinds of parties, dinners, and openings, but rather to know what the twenty-first-century Parisian woman is drinking! Whether in a cocktail bar, club, sidewalk café, luxury hotel coffee shop, fashionable lounge, or wine bar, each has her habits and preferences.

The health-conscious will take the opportunity to have a fresh, antioxidant, anti-aging fruit juice full of vitamins while at the same time maintaining her figure. Not much fun but effective—especially if the aperitif becomes a daily ritual! The traditionalist will order a glass of good wine or

a flute of very cold champagne, absolutely never at room temperature. A critic and connoisseur will ask for the wine list and select her favorite label because she is absolutely forbidden to drink just anything at any temperature! The trend is to drink increasingly dry champagnes such as the very delicate *zéro dosage* (or *brut nature*). There are lovers of *Piscine*—champagne served with a good deal of ice cubes. As a purist with regard to this noble beverage, I tend to consider it sacrilege while recognizing that it is refreshing when drunk outdoors in the summer. The Parisian loves everything that comes from Italy, especially its bubbly sparkling wines. It's very chic to order a *Bellavista Franciacorta Grand Cuvée Satèn* ... in Paris! Or an *Aperol Spritz* with ice cubes and a slice of orange imported from the bars of Venice—the Italian version of the French *Kir Royal.*
The latest trend in Paris is the cocktail, the classic drink

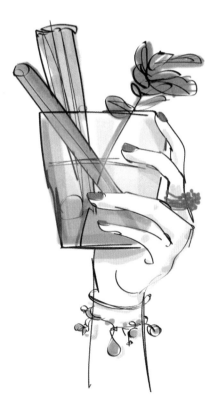

of elderly gentlemen that is now increasingly appreciated by the younger generation. Paris shakes full blast and in every style! Bartenders have become real stars, the grand masters of mixology who create true works of art and who can recommend the right drink for thrill or pleasure and earn the admiration of trendy Parisians. *Grégory Hazac* is one of Parisian women's favorites. Thirty-five years old and the head bartender of the *Hôtel George V* with a brilliant professional career in the most fashionable bars—the *Montecristo Café* in the *Hôtel Costes* and the bars *Royal Monceau* and *Bistrologist*—he added a dose of glamour to the list of Parisian aperitifs by creating the famous *E"V"A Margarita,* a cocktail specially made for Eva Longoria. Another unusual discovery is *Thierry Hernandez*, director of the bar of the *Hôtel Le Bristol,* who asked a couple of years ago *Céline Ellena*, one of the great "noses" of the perfume industry, to create the *Bombay Bahia* cocktail, a recipe that is simultaneously "fire and ice" like the character of a Parisian woman.

Then there are the nostalgic flavors of the past for lovers of retro drinks. The vermouths have been called back into service along with true bitters; there is the great return of the *Bloody Mary* and the *Moscow Mule,* a cocktail created during Prohibition that is based on lime, vodka, and ginger beer.

But for an aperitif, the Parisian woman sips vintage international drinks—*Sazerac, Negroni,* and the *Side Car* are now part of her happy-hour vocabulary.

Attitude

"Parisian women," said Honoré de Balzac, "are inexplicable." Paradox is second nature to them, and they are virtuosos of contradiction. The *Parisienne* is solid and rational but bohemian and insouciant. She's sophisticated yet natural, sexy but lazy, impertinent but discreet. Her hair is immaculately styled yet deliberately tousled. She is the height of chic but wants her look to appear absolutely effortless. Her spirit of contradiction is perhaps part of her unfading charm. She is an ungraspable mystery who "laughs when she is sad and cries when she is happy," as my Italian friend Anna said the other day. Parisian femininity is a blend of different ingredients and condiments: sweet and salty, spicy and suave. But it is not always as it seems: behind the Parisian's paradoxical and changing attitude there is often a good dose of involvement and perfectionism, and that goes for anything she does, starting with her style. Although her look may seem spontaneous, it has

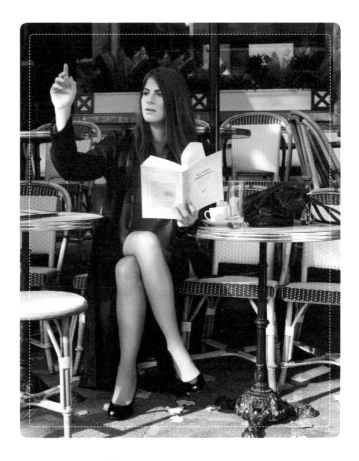

in fact been thoroughly thought out in advance. She knows what looks good on her. She has good taste but creates her own style. She has one eye on the latest fashions and the other on her figure. Her creative spirit builds a look from the "basics" in her wardrobe. She anticipates situations and manages to look natural whatever comes up, in Paris or elsewhere. Invited to a cocktail party at the last moment? She's got the right pair of heels in her bag. An unexpected hot date? She always has chic underclothes on. A bike ride across Paris? It's not her little black dress under her trench coat that will stand in her way!

At the dinner table, the Parisian woman's attitude is a little bit rigid but irreproachable. She sits up straight, with a large napkin spread over her lap and her knees together. Her forearms are properly placed, and she moves slowly and smoothly. She takes small mouthfuls and savors every morsel. Her senses are heightened to fully appreciate the dining experience. Her dinner conversation is cultivated and does not make waves. To some, she is "so chic"; to others she is merely "so cold." Either way, Parisian table manners are an essential part of *savoir-vivre* for any woman who wants to be seen as stylish in the French capital.

Last but not least, the Parisian loves tradition and brings up her children with a sense of values. At the same time, she likes contemporary art and opens the gates of the world to her kids. A fusion attitude!

Avenue Montaigne

Even if the true Parisian woman snobbily claims to belong to the *Rive Gauche* and openly criticizes "the charming idiot" who frequents the *Rive Droite*, the *Avenue Montaigne* in the heart of the so-called Golden Triangle is certainly in her address book! She will do a working lunch, "because she can't do otherwise" at *Avenue* restaurant,

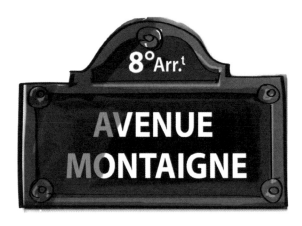

taking advantage of the opportunity to make a fashion run to *Montaigne Market,* the multi-brand luxury store in the district, or to *Chloé, Ungaro, Valentino, Versace, Prada, Armani, Ralph Lauren, D&G, Dior,* or *Nina Ricci.* She will only look because even though she sometimes purchases her basics from the great designers, she tries to buy them at a discount on the first day of a sale. In the evening, elegant in her *petite robe noire* (little black dress), she will go to the *Théâtre des Champs-Elysées* for a concert or to the premiere of one of the major operas of the season and then go to dinner at the *Bar des Théâtres* or the *Relais Plaza,* the Paris meeting point for fashion and business. At nightfall, she will meet her Italian friends at *Chez Francis* for a drink or oysters and a glass of chilled red wine (more chic than white) before the grand spectacle of the lit-up Tour Eiffel. She can even make a dash at lunchtime during the week to see the new arrivals at the luxury outlets in the area. In short, whether for shopping or social life, not a week goes by without taking a trip to the avenue famous for its shops and luxurious gardens surrounded by railings. But *Avenue Montaigne* is much more than a street—it is a concept, a place so famous all over the world that a committee was created on its behalf. Most of the fashion and luxury houses are headquartered there, and it has organized events that punctuate the Parisian social calendar such as the *Election des Catherinettes* and *Art Montaigne*. And don't forget the *Vendanges Montaigne*, the not-to-be-missed event in September, when the luxury houses offer a great wine or champagne to their "super select" clientele.

B

Bag

The Parisian and her bag—a centuries-old love affair. Our bag can be teensy, just large enough for a phone and a credit card. Or it can be humongous, a virtual annex of our home ... we love it!

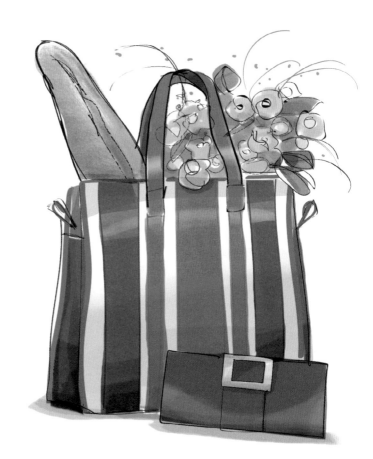

LINKS
- Accessories
- Basic Wear
- Black
- Fashion Shopping

MY TIP
Of course, the main function of a bag is to hold your stuff, but the choice of the right bag for you depends on how you carry it. One doesn't carry an *Un Jour un Sac* tote bag the same way one clutches a *Lady Dior!*

"For busy days we even carry bags in bags, like Russian *matryoshka* dolls. A nice big *Balenciaga* tote bag can hide a *Roger Vivier* evening clutch bag, plus a makeup kit, plus a *Céline* or *Avril Gau* mini sling bag."
Alice, Rue de Condé, January 17

In a nutshell, the Parisian woman is practical. To avoid running back and forth between home, work, kids' school, cocktails at *Café de Flore,* a *vernissage* in Le Marais, and dinner at *La Closerie des Lilas,* she stows everything away in a catchall she calls her purse. Not easy, given that over the week her bag can accumulate kids' report cards, fashion magazines such as *Grazia* to be trendy, an umbrella, a shopping list, a phone charger, the last exhibit catalog of the *Perrotin Galerie,* three packs of tissues, a pair of shoes to take to the cobbler, letters, bills, and oversized *Chloé* glasses, not to mention a jewel cuff to accessorize her *A.P.C.* jacket for a look of aloof Parisian elegance in case an evening requires an extra touch of panache.

• Elbow bag. The Parisian loves to carry her bag like Grace Kelly in the 1950s. But do be careful: the bag shouldn't be so heavy that you get tennis elbow! My favorites include the *Balenciaga City, Lancel French Flair, Agnès B Cabas New York,* the *Longchamp Pliage,* the *Zadig & Voltaire Sunny,* and *Louis Vuitton Speedy,* a fantastic bag for both daily and weekend indispensable items.
• Handbag. A must for every *fashionista!* Part of a classy, slim look, and an essential part of the Parisian wardrobe. There are lots of shapes from which to choose. My favorites: a *Gérard Darel Rebelle,* a *Chloé Paraty,* and a small *Saint-Laurent* tote.
• Sling bag. We love it because it keeps our hands free! A little neglected in recent years, it has resisted the trend of the bag carried in the hand or on the elbow. If you don't want to appear like a student at the Sorbonne but want a fresh and stylish look, choose your bag and your look carefully. My favorites: a small black *Céline,* a *Gérard*

Darel Lipp Léopard, a *Jérôme Dreyfus,* and a *Céline Lefébure.* The 1970s-style flap hobo bag has made a big comeback this year, so time to get yours now!

• Shoulder bag. Feminine par excellence. Never goes out of style. The Parisian loves it in quality fabrics. She'll tend to choose black, brown, or a neutral color that will go with anything. It's an essential, a "basic." By the way, if you're petite, a really big shoulder bag might not suit you.

• Clutch bag. The Parisian slips a clutch into a bigger bag and takes it out for an art opening or an evening downtown. We gals think they're sexy and feminine. Our men, on the other hand, tend to think they're kind of silly. "What's the point," they wonder, "of a bag that can hardly hold a set of keys and an iPhone?" But we love them. They're a convenient way to look more glamorous. They come in all sorts of materials from vinyl to python and every color from black to Klein blue (the iris blue of the famous painter) to orange. Personally speaking, *j'adore*! Do be careful, though, if you're a big woman. Itsy-bitsy bags are not becoming on Amazons.

• Backpack. Why is it that a Parisian will gladly wear a backpack when she's away on vacation, whereas she wouldn't be caught dead wearing one back home in Paris? Ok, backpacks are practical, I'll admit, but a rucksack is not exactly the epitome of refinement and chic. In other words, a pack is just not "my bag"!

Baguette

Une baguette s'il vous plait. Pronouncing these words will get you a fragrant and crunchy loaf of French bread straight from the oven of a Parisian *boulangerie* (bakery). The long, thin loaf called a baguette (literally, "stick") is just as much an emblem of French culture as the Tour Eiffel or the painter Renoir. Not every loaf is worthy of the noble title of baguette, however. There are strict rules: nine ounces of dough, hand-rolled and shaped

LINKS
• Cheese
• Foie gras
• Plating
• Wine

into a thirty-four-inch-long, two-inch-wide loaf with seven notches. Parisians have varied tastes in baguettes and different habits: a traditional baguette for everyday meals, a baguette *briochée* for noshing, and a multigrain or olive baguette for the weekend. There are purists who like a plain baguette spread with lightly salted butter and jam for breakfast, and those who only enjoy it with ripe Normandy *Camembert* cheese and a glass of Bordeaux Saint-Emilion or Saumur Rouge. Gourmets love to dip it in sauce or use it in onion soup recipes. French kids dip it into soft-boiled eggs at dinner or munch it spread with a chocolate paste. Any way it is served, the baguette is

MY TIP

How do you recognize a good baguette? All freshly baked French bread smells mouthwateringly marvelous, so fragrance is not in itself a guarantee of top quality. The baguette par excellence must have a thin, light golden brown crust. The white part of the bread should be cream colored and have a soft, moist consistency, with a slightly nutty aftertaste. My favorite baguettes: *Boulangerie Gontran Cherrier*, Montmartre (18th arrondissement); *Paul*, Saint Germain-des-Prés (6th arrondissement; *Boulangerie Dupain*, Bastille (11th arrondissement).

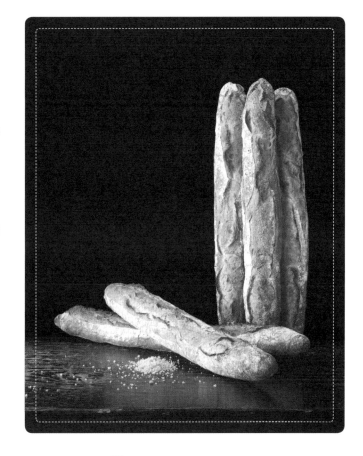

an indispensable part of French life, regardless of age, gender, or milieu. The secret to really enjoying a baguette? As soon as you step out of the bakery, break off one end of the baguette and savor it while it is still crunchy on the outside and soft and warm on the inside. It's doubly delicious if it's hot out of the oven!

Ballerina Shoes

It is said that in Paris, all little girls are born with ballet shoes on their feet! And if that's not the case, as soon as they reach sixth grade their mom takes them to *Bonpoint* to choose their first pair. Then come classical dance lessons, with real ballerina slippers, and the dream of one day starring at the *Opéra de Paris*. As time passes and the little girl becomes a teenager, ballerina shoes become practically a second skin for her. Within a few years she has grown into a young lady, and here she is, running around

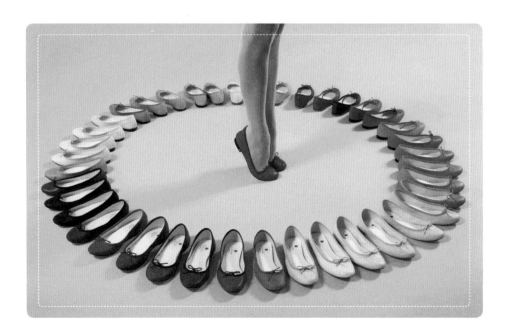

HISTORY

In 1947 Rose Repetto reinvented the dance slipper with a new technique consisting of stitching the sole inside out. In 1956 Brigitte Bardot wore *Repetto* ballerinas in the film *And God Created Woman (Et Dieu . . . créa la femme)* and the fashion became global. Since then, *Lanvin, Chanel, Roger Vivier, Marc Jacob, Inès de la Fressange,* and the other top designers all have their own ballerina model.

the *Ville Lumière*—morning, noon, and night—clad in her ballerinas, her light and comfortable "glass slippers." The young lady has become an authentic, chic *Parisienne*, nonchalant and skilled at playing with contrasts. She's still wearing ballerina shoes, either to reinforce a given look or to attenuate it, depending on her needs, her mood, and her style. In another twenty years or so, her ballerina shoes will have become one of the basic essentials of her wardrobe. But make no mistake: though ballerinas come in every style, color, and quality, the Parisian woman is knowledgeable and has discerning taste. She's not about to wear "just anything." Whether the ballerinas are a designer shoe or a mass-market brand, they must be cut right, have a mini heel (neither too high nor too low), and be made of quality leather.

How to wear them like a Parisian? First, it depends on the clothes. The ballerina shoe looks fresh and pretty with a short trapezoidal or ruffled skirt and a more casual top—maybe a sweater or a *Maje* or *Ba&sh* jacket. Timeless classic footwear in Paris, black ballerinas can be worn with tight skinny jeans or with a knee-length pencil skirt. They also look nice with rolled up chinos, baring the ankle (there's nothing more feminine!), and a beautiful belted low-cut jacket. I wear mine with black *Jitrois* lambskin pants and a white *Eric Bompard* cashmere sweater for a mix of styles: 50% rock 'n' roll, 50% classic charm. Or with one of my little 1950s-style dresses for a vintage look. There are errors of taste that a Parisian never makes, like wearing ballerinas with opaque hose or with a long skirt, baggy slacks, or a pants suit. These combinations somehow tend to make you look "stocky," whereas the Parisian must look slim at all costs.

MY TIP

Choose open-toe-style ballerinas, like the *Cendrillon* model by *Repetto* (photo), the Parisian's favorite brand, or a pair by *Chloé,* which are also very feminine. In the privacy of your own home, you can wear your ballerinas with a baby-doll nightie—so much more sensual and Parisian than wooly socks or Homer Simpson slippers!

Basic Wear

To be honest, I love the basic items of my wardrobe! Since they are the "pillars" that must last over time, they must be of quality, so I choose great designer labels. It's a sort of long-term investment in clothing, garments purchased after strategic reflection and rarely on impulse. Often, I buy my "luxury" basics during sales or at outlet stores or private showrooms reserved for the press.

I also buy quality secondhand clothing, especially black tailored dresses and evening bags. These are garments or accessories (classic models in neutral colors) that follow me everywhere, because they are timeless and easy to wear. When I have to get rid of them because they are too worn or outdated, I often replace them with more or less the same style. They are the basics that prevent opening the closet in the morning and saying: "I have nothing to wear." Among these items there are also shoes (a typically Parisian disease), belts, and scarves.

• Thirteen basic black garments that I would take with me to a desert island: a well-made tuxedo jacket (vintage or contemporary), evening pants to wear with high heels, a pencil skirt (my reference in case of weight gain), a shaped cashmere cardigan (ideal over any evening

LINKS
• Accessories
• Elegance
• Shoes
• Suitcase

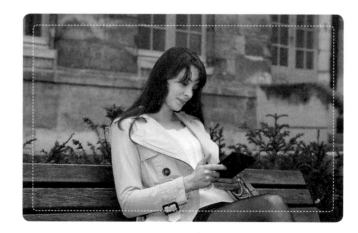

dress), a short schoolgirl skirt (not mini), a cocktail dress "without sparkles," a glamorous and chic long dress, a shaped coat for all occasions, a cashmere stole to use as a shawl or blanket (while watching TV or on an airplane), a beautiful two-piece swimsuit (nice classic model that fits well) and a one-piece swimsuit for water gymnastics and spas, a masculine-shaped jacket, and leather pants in an ultra-classic, feminine style.

• Seven basic blue items of my childhood: a nice pair of dark trousers for all occasions (*Joseph*); an elegant well-cut blazer; a sweater (cashmere, of course); a coat with buttons in a matching color; a striped long-sleeve *marinière* (sailor shirt); a light turtleneck to wear under a jacket in the winter and with white pants on a cool evening in the summer; and jeans, the "good ones"—which is to say, perfect for me.

• My "so French" basic items in light shades: a go-everywhere trench coat (even over an evening gown); stylish white cotton trousers; a white top with a perfect neckline (neither too much nor too little), an ecru cashmere v-neck pullover; an embroidered white cotton tunic that goes with everything in the summer; a shaped white shirt (nice cut and neck); and a white two-piece swimsuit; an ultra-white T-shirt of high quality cotton (blank or with a sober pattern).

• My favorite accessories: low black ballerinas (for all seasons) and a beige pair for spring; high quality "nude look" sandals that I wear like jewels on manicured feet; low black boots (Italian, but don't tell anyone); black moccasins; a pair of patent-leather ballerina shoes with a low heel for the evening; black sandals with a four-inch heel to wear year-round; a big tote bag for the daytime; a black patent-leather clutch for the evening; a black leather belt for pants; a black mini belt for pullovers and jackets; and a pair of oversized dark glasses. And finally: scarves and shawls, caps and hats, and lingerie, especially in black or white lace and some in beige or red.

Bathing Suits

The Parisian woman knows her body and its faults and would die rather than appear vulgar or inadequate. Whether she's wearing a bathing suit or a business suit, it's essential to choose an outfit that makes the most of her assets, detracting attention from her imperfections and adding a touch of style (chic but soft). More than a fashionable or trashy bathing suit, she looks for the perfect shape and a flattering color. There's the Parisian who will only wear *Eres*—expensive but classy, feminine, and timeless. Then there are those who switch from *Etam* to *Banana Moon*, *Princesse Tam Tam*, *Kiwi Saint-Tropez*, *RougeGorge*, *Albertine*, *Pain de Sucre*, and lots of other great French brands. So if you have a picture in your head of a topless Parisian woman on vacation in Saint-Tropez, it's time to think again. Nowadays, whether she's on a beach in Paris (yes, that's right, there's a beach in the city), Brittany, the southwest, the Côte d'Azur or even sunbathing on a boat, she will always be relaxed and confident. She loves "beautiful bathing suits," by which I mean real swimsuits, made up of a top, a bottom, and possibly a wrap or cover-up for the sushi and cocktails break.

Unless your name is Cara Delevingne, Constance Jablonski, or Thylane Blondeau, it's hard to find a two-piece bathing suit in which both the top and the bottom fit perfectly. Look for brands that offer the chance to choose the size and style of each piece.

• Choose the model then the pattern, not the other way round.

• The shape of the top depends on your breasts! This isn't something new, yet it seems to cause a problem every time. Whether you have a generous bosom or are completely flat, the choice of the right top is fundamental. For medium breasts, an unpadded *balconette* style is always elegant and sensual, and creates a natural bosom. For small breast to avoid looking too boyish, prefer super-feminine models but without too much padding—otherwise they could end up

MY TIP
The Parisian's secret? Simple: to be elegant, she chooses one understated, good quality suit (rather than four patterned medium-quality suits); to be comfortable and natural, she chooses a style that flatters her figure, looks good, and allows her to relax rather than focus on her complexes. In short, she picks a bathing suit that suits her size (neither too large nor too small), her shape, and the color of her skin. Nothing colorful. The Parisian prefers the basics—a black or a bright white two-piece, a black or a navy one-piece. Patterns (gingham checks, flowers, ethnic-chic, or colors) come second.

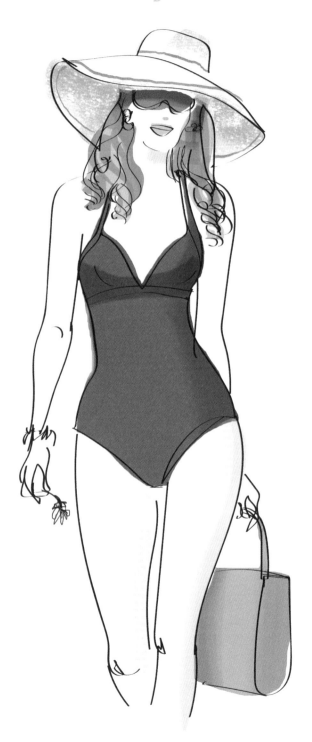

looking fake. For a generous bosom, look for that rare jewel that will support and contain your breasts properly (with reinforcing and broad straps in the right place, not too far apart). The push-up, to be used with moderation, is fine for breasts that are far apart, because it brings them closer together, creating a natural volume. Be careful with bandeau styles, though, because not all breasts look good in tops that squash them or allow them to sag. They're nice and practical but better if you choose them with built-in cups and ties to knot behind your neck. Be critical when you look in the mirror. Take a close look then stand back, look at the details, turn around ...

• The shape of the bottom depends on the width of your hips, your buttocks, and your thighs. If you are petite, with slender hips and flat buttocks, prefer styles with frills, bows, or decorations—pearls or rings on the sides or with textured effects. That will add some necessary volume. Mini styles with a high-cut leg will also make you look more feminine, accentuating your hips. If you have big rounded hips, try not to draw attention to them—choose a very plain bottom, avoiding those with a low rise, in order to draw the eye upward with a good top. A hipster/boxer style is the big-hipped woman's best friend, while the string is her worst enemy! And naturally, avoid anything too small that would create rolls and bulges.

• For larger ladies, the best style is the one-piece, with the lower part as plain as possible and an attractive v-neck or draped neckline. This year, the one-piece is really fashionable, so take advantage. Glamorous and elegant at the same time, it's no longer reserved for women over fifty or oversized. And it's fine for the beach, not just for exercising at the pool. The only problem is that after two weeks at the beach, you'll find yourself with a bright white tummy! But the experts are certain that "this type of style allows you to enhance your figure, hiding any hipline bulges." If you really must have a two-piece, do like the large Parisian, her mother, and her grandmother, and opt for high-waist bottoms: very 1940s!

Beach

In summer, the Parisian heads for the sea, spending her vacations in Brittany, in the family home on the Île de Ré (or the super chic Île d'Yeu), or in southwest France (Arcachon, Biarritz, Cap Ferret ...), Normandy, or the Côte d'Azur. This is when Paris is overtaken by tourists. The city is hot, the fountains are mobbed by tourists, and the desire for the beach and the sea is strong. And that's fine, because the *Ville Lumière* has its very own sandy beaches along the banks of the River Seine. Obviously, you cannot go for a dip the way you can in Deauville or Saint-Tropez, but you can build sandcastles under the palms, sunbathe on a deckchair, and relax under umbrellas the way you would by the sea but right in the center of Paris! This incredible, fun attraction is something to experience,

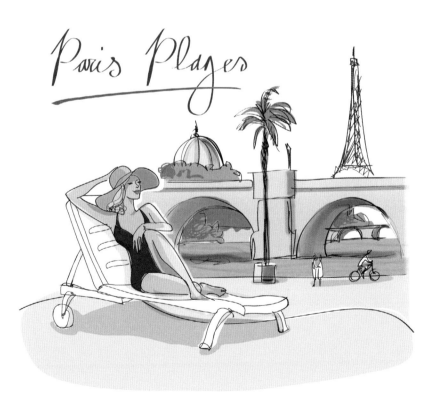

Paris Plages

or at least to see, between July and mid-August. Two miles of the road along the river are closed to traffic and set up for tourists and the few Parisians that are still in the city. It is the most intriguing and enjoyable form of summer entertainment in Paris. For more information, see the Tourist Office website. See you at the Paris *plage* next summer.

Bicycle

"At the weekend, getting out on our bikes offers us a different view of Paris, taking in the quiet districts and secluded corners that are hard to reach by car. In the evening, when the last *métro* has gone and you can't get a cab, we have no problem climbing on a bike and cycling home, regardless of what we're wearing and how high our heels are."
Barbara, Place des Vosges, March 16

Cycling in Paris is fun, and riding around on a bike offers Parisian women the chance to combine business with pleasure, in a manner of speaking; forget about the traffic, everyday stress, and worries; and get some exercise on their way to work or to an appointment. Even the little black dress adapts to the situation! It's fun to see all these elegant women pedaling around Paris, admiring monuments, buildings, and beautifully lit bridges. The city

MY TIP
In *Paris*, your *vélo* (the bike) is a real vehicle, for all intents and purposes, which is why it's essential to respect the local laws—for your safety and that of others. For example, you cannot cycle on sidewalks or with your cell phone in your hand, and you cannot chain your bike to a public structure outside the reserved spaces. It is best to use the cycle paths and give way to pedestrians crossing the road. And most important of all: pay attention to the sudden opening of the doors of parked cars, as this was the cause of more than one hundred accidents in Paris! Make sure you can be seen at night! Fit a light to the front of your bike and one to the back and add some reflectors. Enjoy your ride!

LINKS
• Grayness
• Sky
• Sunset
• Walk in Paris

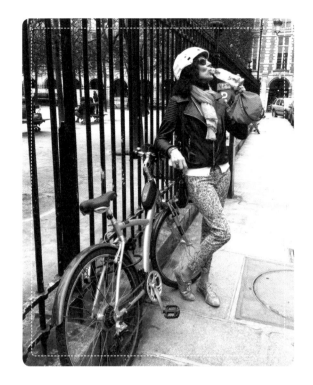

is fantastic by night! But very few Parisians actually have their own bike. They generally use the *Vélib'* (24/7 bike sharing with stations installed by the City Council all over Paris). I highly recommend them for getting off the beaten track and exploring the Parisians' Paris.

When I have time, I take a quick look around the Rive Gauche (Left Bank). Are you tempted? Starting at the *Jardins des Plantes,* head toward the Institut du Monde Arabe then the Panthéon (watch out for the climb), the Jardins du Luxembourg, the Sénat (senate), Place Saint-Sulpice (for a glimpse of the church), Rue du Cherche-Midi (shopping), the Musée d'Orsay, the Invalides (a picnic on the grass), and the Quai Branly (also a museum), and end up at the Tour Eiffel. You can then cross over to the Rive Droite (Right Bank) and continue through the evening …

Bidet

HISTORY
History does not recall if there was a Mr. Bidet. There are various stories about the birth of the bidet ... It was invented in the seventeenth century for the royal French family and later became famous in houses of ill repute. By the time the last brothel in France was closed, in 1946, the image of the bidet had become so tainted by that of the cathouse that many French women were prejudiced against using it.

If the word *bidet* is part of my book, it is because I find it one of the more paradoxical words in the French language. The bidet was invented in France three centuries ago and then exported to the four corners of the earth. The paradox is that though the bidet is quintessentially French, there is nary a bidet to be found in Paris these days! Because they take up too much room for a modern Parisian bathroom (which is smaller than forty-five square feet), bidets started to disappear in the 1970s, and it's now difficult to find one in a modern apartment or in a hotel in the French capital! When asked, "How do you manage without a bidet?" Parisians reply:

"We take something called a shower!"
Colette, Place Pompidou, January 8

"We take a 'full-body' approach to cleanliness rather than washing one bit at a time!"
Manon, Rue Bizet, April 5

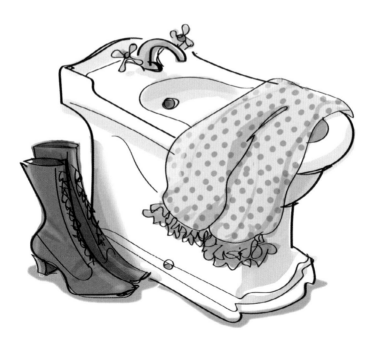

Among the few hotels in Paris today that have a bidet are the *Atlantic, Caravelle, Champs-Élysées Plaza, Darcet, Four Seasons George V, Lancaster, Magellan,* and *Le Meurice.*

Bistro

LINKS
- Cafés
- Friendship
- Gratin
- Wine

If the letter B is often associated with Brigitte Bardot, in Paris it takes on all its *grandeur* at the beginning of the word *bistro.* It is an institution, a universally recognized and appreciated word, synonymous with informal gastronomy. A magical place where the Parisian woman loves to spend the evening with her friends or

MY TIP
There are so many bistros in Paris that the Parisian woman has difficulty choosing and, above all, not making a mistake! That is why she always has at hand a restaurant guide and the *Lebey* bistro guide, the reference book on the subject. The best way to know the best bistros of the year is to read the critics that write for Parisians and not for tourists!

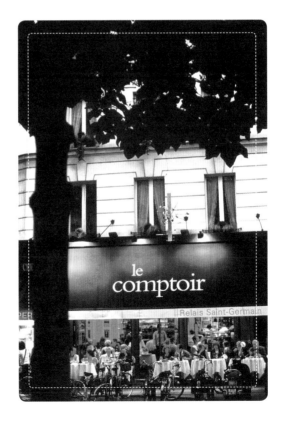

HISTORY
In the 1990s, tempted by the bistro experience, some of the great Parisian chefs opened places—true "annexes" of their gastronomic restaurants—offering their fans a simpler, more everyday cuisine, using less expensive products but prepared with gastronomic inspiration. The "Bistrot-Gastro" was born. "Refinement, friendliness, and reasonable prices," a boon for lovers of good food! My favorites: Christian Constant's *Café Constant,* Guy Savoy's *Bouquinistes,* Pierre Gagnaire's *Gaya,* and, of course, Yves Camdeborde's *Comptoir du Relais.* The dishes are gourmet but light. Incredibly modern food for the Parisian who loves to eat but wants to stay slim.

her husband. And when the bistro is combined with gastronomy, it gives birth to "bistronomy" to the great delight of the capital's gourmets, who, in a more casual atmosphere, can enjoy a meal made with local products and traditional recipes prepared at more affordable prices than those of the great starred restaurants.

Bocca Rossa, Mensae and *L'Agrume* are some of the Parisian restaurants I like the best these days, but my top favorite is still *Les Enfants Rouges,* in the historic district of Le Marais. The cuisine there is so delicate, a paradoxical mix of rustic and luxury foods. Chef Daï Shinozuka, formerly with Yves Camdeborde's famous *Le Comptoir du Relais* bistro, reinvents French cuisine with Japanese inspiration. Shinozuka's amazing dishes are as pleasing to the eye as they are to the palate. Simplified traditional French recipes sublimed with the flavors of Japan. With perfect technique and great imagination, the chef creates ingenious flavorful twenty-first-century cuisine. Also noteworthy, *Firmin le Barbier* is a tiny but super nice bistro on a side street of the 7th arrondissement with a view of the Tour Eiffel in the front. It is known for creative recipes with top quality products. For fine modern bistro cuisine, try the *Roca* restaurant in the 17th arrondissement. Alexandre Giesbert is a master of technique and quality, who learned from top Parisian chefs including Pierre Gagnaire and Éric Briffard. Surprisingly creative cooking, especially the blends of tastes and textures.

Another good address: *A. Noste,* Rue du 4 Septembre. Fantastic, hearty, generous, tasty Basque cooking; a mixture of country-style and city-style cuisine.

It's not only the customers that dream of fashionable Parisian bistros. Talents from all over the world are now coming to try their own gourmet bistro formulas. Japanese, British, and Italian chefs are bringing their touch of genius to Parisian "bistronomy." My favorite: Massimiliano Alajmo (a Michelin three-star chef in Italy) at the *Caffè Stern,* in the beautiful Passage des Panoramas. Here you will find dishes with character.

Brilliant contemporary renditions of Venetian classics.
I recommend *dill tagliolini*. Simply superb! Or savor
Venetian-style liver with crispy polenta ... Enjoy it with
some nice *Barbaresco* or *Barolo* wine! I am crazy about
involtini di scampi fritti con salsa di bottarga.

Black

Black is the Parisian woman's color. Beyond the boulevard
périphérique—the wall that "protects" the capital—women
wear beige, blue, and pastel tones, but in the *Ville Lumière*,
black persists and always wins.
Although the runways and fashion magazines offer
the new colors of the season, when buying, reason beats

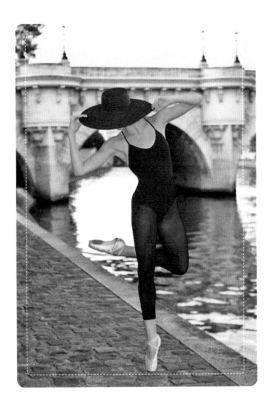

LINKS
• Bag
• Red
• Vintage
• Wardrobe

HISTORY
Once upon a time, black was the color of "princes" because it was austere but elegant; then it became the symbol of sophisticated evening dresses dear to Coco Chanel and tuxedos by Yves Saint-Laurent. Today it is the symbol of absolute modern elegance; black is the Parisian woman's uniform.
In contrast to aggressive and pompous colors, it can emphasize character and conversation, like the frame of a painting, or otherwise allow you to blend into the crowd. The choice is yours!

emotion and the *Parisienne* chooses black because it is the "master key" that goes with everything and suits all situations.

The Parisian just changes accessories to create a new look and goes from flats to a *décolleté* with a four-inch stiletto heel, from "nude" makeup to scarlet lipstick, adds a cardigan to her little black dress from the office and is immediately ready for an evening look. Black is infinitely adjustable. Even black underwear sells better than white or flesh-colored in Paris! It is a safe bet, a guaranteed investment because it is timeless.

In the end, we always go back to black because the Parisian is rational and likes clothing that lasts—not ephemeral one-season garments. And then, color requires good taste, and the risk of clashing discourages more than a few, because Paris has difficulty accepting vulgarity, even if creative! Bright colors are often limited to accessories, handbags, and scarves to give a touch of fun or to enliven a too sober look. Plus, in black, a fabric of inferior quality or an inadequate model, can go unnoticed, but in orange it would be really terrible.

Blue

Blue—navy blue—is the favorite color of the *Parisienne*— after black, of course! Perhaps it's because it makes her think about vacations? It gives her a feeling of escape and open spaces? It evokes a "cruise" look, symbolic of getting away from the gray of winter? It reminds her of her childhood school? Or simply because blue, ever since Yves Saint-Laurent introduced it in his collections combined with black, has become the epitome of chic? In effect, blue is super stylish, goes well with everything, and is "cool" to the right point! What Parisian woman doesn't have a blue sweater in her closet ever since the 1980s, when she listened a thousand times to the song *Pull marine*, written by Serge Gainsbourg for Isabelle Adjani? Whatever the

LINKS
• Black
• Red
• Wardrobe

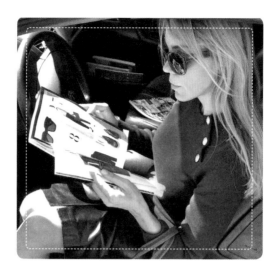

reason, it's good to wear everywhere because it is said that blue "has a calming effect." In spring, blue is everywhere—in shop windows, on the terraces of cafés, in the street. Except for the lack of boats and the sea, Paris seems like a seaside resort!

Bride

Forget the meringue-shaped colored dress, "carnival" makeup, frizzy chignons, and bouquets too full of decorative accessories. The Parisian bride is delicate, feminine, or sensual but, above all, never "tacky." The trendy and poetic romantic wears a bohemian-style dress with a simple but studied high-fashion line inspired by the 1920s with a few ornaments, lace, embroidery, or mother-of-pearl buttons and a little crown of beautiful wildflowers. The current trend is vintage revisited. The glamour bride opts for a tight-fitting model to which she adds a risqué note: a deep back is very current (an exuberant femininity, a bride to make your head spin). In Parisian churches, we are seeing a great return of the veil, in the long or short

LINKS
• Accessories
• Class
• Lingerie
• Wardrobe

MY TIP
As a rule, don't use too many accessories; elegance can also be simple—only one or two accessories rather than three or four. You have to look cool and chic, not as if you were going to a masquerade ball. Study your bouquet well. It shouldn't be too heavy (think about your girlfriends when you throw it) or too perfumed. It should be well prepared so the flowers do not fall, wilt, or stain your dress.

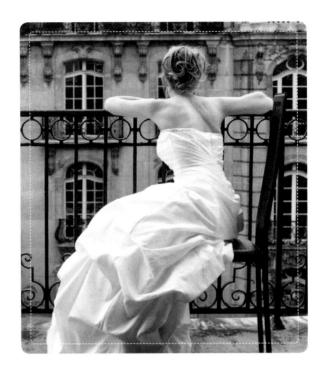

and light version. *Très chic!* In any case, even if the important thing is the emotional "hit," don't forget that you will have to like how you look in thirty years, when you look at your wedding photo on the piano in the living room. And remember: "The most beautiful bride is the one that remains true to herself."
Follow these simple rules and you will be the perfect bride:

• Avoid choosing a dress or a hairstyle that doesn't suit you. You will do well to reflect for a moment. Think of elegance, of the pictures, and the comments of your friends.

• Think about your desires and the bride you want to be. Search the Internet for dresses from the big names to see the models, even if you opt for your local seamstress. Go see a lot of dresses before trying them on to refine your taste. And, above all, take your time.

- Avoid playing designer by combining the neckline of one stylist with the sleeves of another and the veil of a third—the result is extremely risky.
- Choose a dress appropriate to the style of the wedding: for a chic wedding, classic elegance is *de rigueur*; in a dance hall on the banks of the Seine, a 1950s dress will be more suitable.
- Take a dress that fits well on the day you try it on—not too small. Just tell the seamstress of your intention to lose five pounds and she will adjust the dress in due time, if necessary.
- Forget the chic lingerie under a wedding dress and pick something in microfiber, the color of your skin and without seams.

Bridges

The bridges in Paris are much more than just a way of getting from one bank of the Seine to the other; they're a distinct part of Parisian life. Each one has its own story, atmosphere, and life ... like all Parisian women. I love and adore them. Here's a little song about bridges.

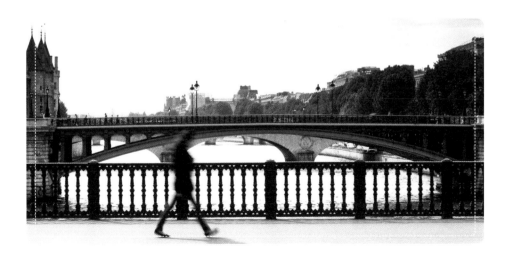

The Wind, by Georges Brassens

If by chance,
on the Pont des Arts
you meet the wind, the cheeky wind,
be prudent, watch out for your skirt!
If by chance,
on the Pont des Arts
you meet the wind, the rascal wind,
be cautious, watch out for your hat!

Fools and the well-bred
speak ill of the furious wind
that uproots trees,
blows off roofs,
lifts skirts ...
But fools and the well-bred
I assure you, mean nothing
to the wind, and he's right!

If by chance,
on the Pont des Arts,
you meet the wind, the cheeky wind,
be prudent, watch out for your skirt!
If by chance,
on the Pont des Arts,
you meet the wind, the rascal wind,
be cautious, watch out for your hat!

Of course, if your opinion is based
solely on what you see with your eyes,
the wind appears to be a brute who enjoys
harming all he sees ...
But a deeper analysis
reveals that he prefers to choose pains-in-the-ass
as the victims of his tricks!

C

Cafés

It's hard to imagine Paris without cafés! Bars, cafés, taverns, and bistros vary according to cultural heritage, but the principle remains the same: a convivial place where you laugh, chat, change the world, read the newspaper, listen to the latest gossip, and maybe give a final touch to a document on your computer before a meeting. The Parisian woman loves the relaxed atmosphere and warmth of a café. For her it's a place to meet others or for private relaxation, where she can also enjoy a light meal with her girlfriends at a table or at the counter. In good weather, she prefers an outdoor table, *en terrasse*, to write a few lines, smoke a cigarette, and soak up some sun with her chin lifted upward.

Parisian waiters have a worldwide reputation for being rude, but isn't that what makes them attractive? Imagine a courteous, smiling, and talkative waiter who doesn't limit himself to his few dry and hard words.

MY TIP
The price of what in Paris is called *un petit noir* is far from being the same everywhere and, depending on the neighborhood and the type of place, can be five times as expensive! The Parisian average is about $1.25. But who says a cup of coffee has to be twice as expensive to be twice as good? And, in the end, what does the coffee matter? It's the company that counts.

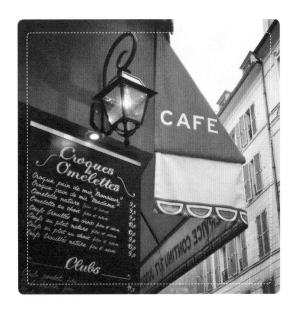

"What'll you have?"
"Are you done? I have to free up the table."
"The toilet? In back to the left."
"Can I collect?"
"I speak only French."
"A coffee, that's all?"
The verbal communication of a Parisian waiter is
relatively limited, but his glance is full of innuendos
that speak volumes:
"Of course, I have nothing else to do."
"I have customers who are waiting for the table."
"I certainly don't make a living from your coffee."
"No tip?"

Champagne

LINKS
• Aperitif
• Gastronomy
• Marianne
• Wine

Good champagne evokes an endless source of emotions.
The Parisian woman's beverage par excellence,
it's also the inevitable tipple for urban diners. Sometimes
it's a bit over the top, because there's not a party when
the hostess doesn't bring out the champagne. This
excessive consumption has generated the production
of a multitude of lower quality champagnes and
generalized the consumption of the planet's most
prestigious beverage, a drink that should remain a symbol
of celebration, luxury, and special occasions.
The Parisian knows how to tell a good champagne
from an ordinary one; she's very critical and loves to give
her opinion. You, too, can learn to recognize what
you're drinking.
• How to recognize quality? The bubbles must be small,
rise in continuous columns from the bottom of the glass,
and not be aggressive on the mouth. The phrase we use
is that the bubbles "tickle the tongue."
The texture of champagnes produced according
to the traditional method should offer a certain density,
due to their long aging process. Try to imagine you've got

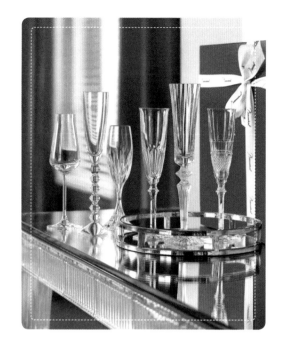

a kind of fabric under your tongue: is it velvet, silk satin, or *crêpe de Chine*?

• Ice in champagne, or not? What we call a *Piscine*— champagne that has become a "swimming pool"—is in at the fashionable places of Paris, a pretentious trend that goes against the grain and lacks sophistication. At *Krug*, for example, once the blend is decided, you have to wait six years before drinking the *Grande Cuvée*, and, when it's a vintage, the wait can be up to fourteen years! Would you want to put an ice cube in this precious drink when it could have taken on the taste of the spinach in your freezer?

• At what temperature should Champagne be served? For fresh young champagnes, serve well chilled between 43°F and 47°F, which will allow the bouquet to develop better and maintain the bubbles; for mature or vintage champagnes, serve between 50°F and 54°F.

• What's the difference between brut and extra brut? The

first has more sugar while the second is almost "pure,"
so it's less sweetened, more mineral—very popular
at the moment.
• Why put salt in the champagne ice bucket? Salt prevents
water from freezing at 32°F (making it freeze at a slightly
lower temperature), so salted ice cubes are slightly colder,
which ultimately means more uniform cooling
of the bottle.
• What stemware to use? Do you prefer a flute or a tulip-
shaped glass? The traditional bowl with its wide opening
has the disadvantage of diffusing the bubbles too quickly
and letting the aromas escape. Champagne is above all
a wine to be inhaled and savored. Silver cups—though
giving a pleasing, fresh contact and with all due respect
for those who love them—are not ideal for consuming
champagne, because they conceal the color and the
perlage of the drink.

Cheese

From the sweetest to the strongest and from the freshest
to the most pasteurized, you can easily find all French
cheeses in Paris—some say more than four hundred
varieties. The choice is huge and everyone can find his
or her own—the important thing is to choose well. So
whether you go, like the elite of Parisian society,
to *Barthélemy* in the 7th arrondissement, *Virginie*
in Montmartre, or even the *très chic Grande Épicerie
de Paris,* get advice. A good cheese vendor is also
a craftsman who knows cheeses perfectly—their
production seasons, their origins, the producers, and
the aging techniques. He has to give honest advice and
convey his love for this product. Living just a short walk
from Saint-Germain market, I am a big fan of *Michel
Sanders,* who has, among others, a Saint-Félicien to make
your head spin and a nice selection of aged Comté,
in a very nice shop. Each year the "Meilleur Ouvrier de

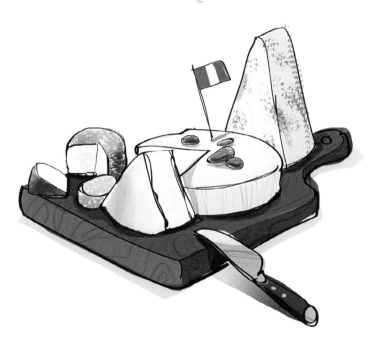

France" (*MOF*) competition names the best craftsmen of the profession, who love their work and have encyclopedic knowledge. Even if Paris is full of good places, Parisians love all that is "the best of." For my part, I love walking to *Laurent Dubois (MOF 2000)* on boulevard Saint-Germain or to *Marie-Anne Cantin*, cheese-seller to the stars, near the Tour Eiffel. For information, the latter organizes educational tastings so you can become familiar with the families of cheeses, their history, their peculiarities, and how to present them, cut them, and preserve them. Increasingly, we often reduce the huge gap between mass-produced and farm (*fermier*) or craft (*artisanal*) cheeses too much. Here are two interesting things to know before buying a cheese, and I leave you to judge what's best for you. Farm cheeses are made with milk from the producer's livestock and processed immediately; craft cheeses are generally produced with milk from many farms in the same region; mass-produced cheeses, sold in supermarkets, are produced with milk from several regions.

MY TIP
In Paris, at a tasting, restaurant, or among friends, etiquette requires that you never, ever touch the cheese with your fingers. Hold it with a piece of bread and cut the crust with a knife. Never use a fork, even if they give you one!

Aging: it is necessary to distinguish between sellers who are supplied by local producers and who then do the aging in their own cellars, and those who buy their cheeses already aged.

A true cultural landmark, cheese is inseparable from everyday life in Paris. A good meal always ends with cheese, a golden rule for Parisian hostesses. A Frenchman may consume more than fifty-five pounds of it per year! At the top of the list are goat cheeses and the good old Camembert, appreciated for its taste but also for its "powerful" emanations! Every region, every city, and every village in France proudly produces its own cheese. In addition, you'll be pleased to know that the current passion of Parisian women is Italian cheeses; we have become great connoisseurs of Parmesan, Pecorino, Burrata, and Mozzarella, which we call "Mozza."

Children

Parisian women grumble that they have no faith in the future and grouse that they no longer trust their institutions. But that doesn't stop them from having plenty of kids! Whereas our neighbors are attempting to check the decline in fertility in order to limit the aging of their populations and the costs that implies, in France a two-child family is considered "classic" and families with three or four kids are commonplace. It is true that France has a longstanding family policy and a tradition of universal child support benefits called *allocations familiales*. But it would appear that culture is the preponderant influence. Family is sacred and the larger family is praised. What's more, French society has never criticized (at least, not too much …) women who entrust their children to nannies or daycare centers. Women with two kids can go back to work and reconcile a career with the joys of motherhood. Today, Parisians tend to have no more than two children.

LINKS
• Eating Right
• Grandma
• Museum
• Parenting

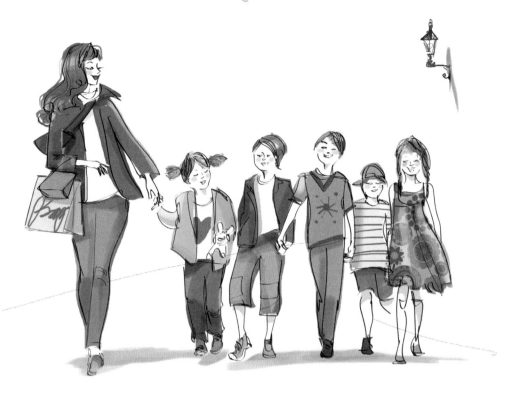

Living is expensive here, and needless to say, Parisian moms want only the best for their little darlings. With just two kids, it's easier to invest in their future so that they can find the most rewarding jobs later on. What's more, with a smaller family, it's easier for a mother to find the right work-life balance without having to make too many concessions: raising children, life as a couple, career, cultural activities, volunteer work, social life, fitness classes and more. Trying to juggle all of that and still look charming and elegant is no easy feat!

Chocolate

This is nothing new—the *Parisienne* loves chocolate. Chocolate in bars, creams, drinks, or creations of master *chocolatiers* such as *Jean-Paul Hévin*, *Pierre Hermé*, and

Hugo & Victor. She's a chocoholic! In tearooms, the star is hot chocolate; in pastry shops, macaroons or chocolate éclairs. And then there is the supermarket, where she buys her bars by the dozen. For twenty years, Paris has hosted the *Salon du Chocolat*, the largest worldwide event dedicated to this product and cocoa! But despite everything, the chocolate-eating Parisian woman is thin? Well, yes, because we especially love rich dark chocolate with 70% cocoa or more, which contains little added sugar and virtually no milk. Doctors say that chocolate can be seamlessly integrated into our daily diet because it is not fattening itself and is excellent for our health. Of course, everything depends on the amount consumed, the frequency of consumption, and the rest of your diet. In any case, chocolate puts you in a good mood, is a natural stress reducer, decreases sleepiness, and increases your attention span and concentration! In addition, it is good for the heart and brain. It is rich in potassium, copper, magnesium, and iron. This is why the Parisian woman jumps on chocolate bars, is the queen of chocolate mousse, and loves the black chocolate creams of *Jacques Genin*, the truffles of *Patrick Roger,* and the chocolate and fresh fruit bars of *Jean-Charles Rochoux*, without forgetting the dark chocolate

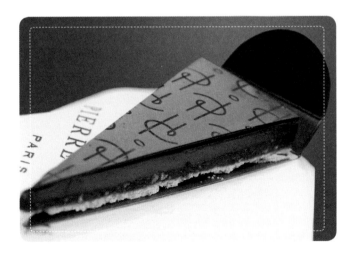

THE RECIPE

*Every Parisian woman
has her own version
of soufflé. This is mine,
made with chocolate.
As for savory soufflés,
I adore the traditional
kind made from cheese,
but I often flavor
it with squid ink ...
Besides being good, it's
beautiful to see: all gray
in a white bowl.*

Chocolate Soufflé

Serves 8

*1 1/2 cup heavy cream
1 1/5 cup semi-sweet chocolate with 70% cocoa, chopped into pieces
1 cup sugar
2 tbsp. corn flour
1 1/2 tbsp. cocoa
8 egg yolks, 8 egg whites
butter for the molds, powdered sugar*

In a bowl add the heavy cream, the cocoa and corn flour after sifting, and bring to a boil, stirring to thicken. Add the chopped up chocolate and the egg yolks, beating constantly. Beat the egg whites until soft peaks are formed; delicately fold in 1/3 of the sugar at the beginning, then 1/3 midway through, and the last 1/3 at the end to make the mixture compact (don't overbeat, the beaten egg whites should be smooth).

Use a silicone or wooden spatula to gradually fold the beaten egg whites into the chocolate mixture, stirring until there is no trace of the egg whites. Butter the soufflé molds twice: grease the mold and refrigerate; then brush the greased mold with melted butter and refrigerate again. Sprinkle lightly with sugar. Delicately pour the mixture into the molds all the way up to the rim. The twice-buttered molds can be refrigerated for up to about 5 hours; they can even be prepared a day or two before and kept in the freezer. In this case they should be removed from the freezer 4-5 hours before cooking. Bake in the oven at 350°F for about 15-20 minutes. Sprinkle lightly with powdered sugar and serve at once.

Note: when I serve my guests soufflé, I accompany it with vanilla ice cream. This dessert is ideal for chocolate-lovers, but even more appreciated at the end of a light meal. It's also easy to make and freeze, so you'll always have it on hand. As for the size of the molds: small molds for individual servings are better than one large mold. The results are better because it's much harder to get a larger mass of soufflé to rise. There are two ways to keep the soufflés well risen: cook them with a firebrick in the oven and, once you've removed the soufflés from the oven, place the firebrick under the mold to maintain the heat: it's the cold-warm contrast that will make a soufflé fall. Or, you can add to the number of egg whites for the recipe, but that will change the flavor, which would be a pity ... Perhaps the best solution is to eat the soufflés right away!

candies filled with almond pralines of *Pierre Marcolini*! But remember that chocolate is high in fat; so, yes, eat it, but focus on quality over quantity. *Less is more*!

Christmas

Parisian women are more conservative than they would have you believe—especially when it comes to memories of childhood and of *l'art de vivre*. Christmas is our childhood, a family tradition that we try to carry on today with our children ...
My Christmas memories ...
"In two days it's Christmas! Paris has been getting ready for three weeks. From the Christmas lights on the Champs-Elysées to elaborate window displays at the capital's most famous department stores, everything is magical and enchanting. 'It's mahvelous, dahling!' said my mom. My name's Emmie. I rewrote my letter to Santa Claus five times. It's not that I changed the toys on my list, it's just that I couldn't find the right words to get him to stop at my house so that I could give him a hug and we could talk. Dad said he had a lot of work on Christmas Eve and that he stopped by for a brief moment. Today, my folks and me and my sisters are driving out to the country to spend Christmas with Grandma 'n Grandpa. I've been dreaming of this trip for a whole year. Apart from the cold, we have such a good time: the riddles and giggles in the car; seeing my cousins again; and playing hide-and-seek in the vineyard. There's all the excitement of the Christmas preparations: my aunts talking for hours, planning Christmas dinner; Grandpa perched on a ladder putting the final touches on the Christmas tree; Grandma cheerfully humming Christmas carols as she sets up the little Nativity scene.
December 24. After church, we all have supper. The grownups have foie gras, which I think is kind of yucky, and oysters (even yuckier!) We kids have crêpes! All

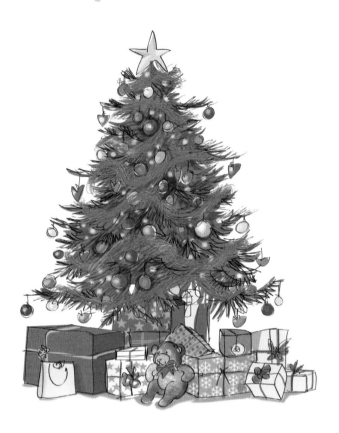

sorts with all sorts of colors: with chocolate past, whipped cream, blueberries, or bananas. Yum! Anyway, it's getting late and the grownups all say they have a lot of work to do, which I don't really understand, but there are so many mysterious things about Christmas. After supper, we all leave a shoe under the Christmas tree for Santa Claus to fill. I put a bright red shoe, because it's really easy to spot, in case Santa is nearsighted like my cousin Eléonore. Florin writes his name in giant letters in case Santa doesn't recognize his shoe, and Gaspard cheats by leaving an après-ski boot (he's noticed that Grandpa, with the biggest shoes in the family, always seems to get the most presents). Grandma sings out: 'Okay, off to bed, kids.' They say, 'Be a good girl and go to sleep. Tonight, Santa Claus is coming, he's gonna come down the chimney and

maybe bring you a present.' Who could believe that? Santa
Claus has too much to carry to fit down the chimney, and
how's he gonna get past the fire? Grandpa always burns
grapevine branches that shoot off sparks like fireworks.
This year, I'm finally gonna solve the mystery ... At last, it's
time to kiss everyone nighty-night. Thirty pecks, smacks,
and smooches later, it's bedtime for me and my kid sister
Jade. I'm sleepy but I'm so excited. Tonight, I'm finally
going to meet Santa Claus in person. Jade is fast asleep.
I slide out of bed and listen by the stairway. There's still
noise in the house. The grownups downstairs are doing
the dishes and getting something ready. I can't figure out
what. They're laughing a lot and seem very busy. I put
on the white dress I wear for special occasions and slip
quietly into the living room. The Christmas tree decorated
by Grandpa stands alone with a ring of shoes around it.
I sit down at the foot of the tree and wait. Maybe if I sing
a song to Santa, he'll come sooner?

'Little Father Christmas, when you come down from the
sky, with toys by the thousands, don't forget my little shoe.
But before leaving, you must cover yourself well, outside
you will be so cold ...'
I'm so sleepy. My lids get heavy and I doze off. I wake up
with a jolt when I hear: 'Little Father Christmas, when you
come down from the sky.' It's Grandma going from room
to room, waking up all the kids singing *Petit Papa Noel*
by Tino Rossi and saying, 'Come on kids! Santa's been
here!! Come on now, everyone up!'
Impossible!!! What happened? Did he leave me a note?
No one seems to know my secret, except maybe Mom,
who says sleeping at the foot of the Christmas tree is not
a sensible thing to do, since a child could catch cold! It's
not funny. Now I'll have to wait a whole 'nother year! Oh,
well! Let's go help Grandma get all the sleepyheads out of
bed so we can finally go into the living room and see what
Santa has brought!
Four years ago, I was the littlest kid, and so I got to go

into the living room first on Christmas morning. This year there are at least eight kids ahead of me. It's no fun getting old! At last Grandpa opens the room, and what a surprise! Baby Jesus is lying in the manger and our shoes are full of gifts! Santa Claus was here but had no time to stop. Once again, it's Grandpa who gets the most presents! I'm a tiny bit disappointed but so happy to see everyone laugh and play!

And Grandma sings and laughs! Thanks Grandma!"

Class

Parisian women are said to have class. Is class a gift? Parisian women are also said to be haughty, arrogant, and snobbish. Perhaps aloof would be a better word. Aloofness may in fact be our way of preserving our privacy. Or could aloofness be a genetically or culturally programmed behavior? Of course, we're proud of belonging to the elite

LINKS
• Attitude
• Elegance
• Grandma
• Vintage

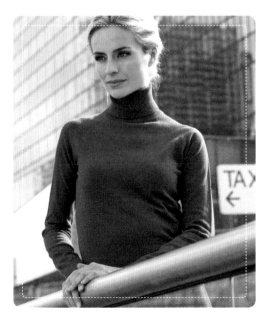

MY TIP

Class is not simply a question of dressing the part. It's also about meticulous attention to your overall look and developing allure and presence. No matter what your weight or budget, anyone can have class. Above all, concentrate on your posture—how you hold your head and the way you walk. Next, without forcing it or going overboard, work on good manners and courtesy. Finally, if you want to achieve a Parisian look, adopt a slightly stuck-up air of nonchalance; the height of class is that it has to appear unconscious and effortless.

Remember that everything about you should appear natural, including your presence, which should generate an aura of discreet strength.

who reside in the *Ville Lumière*, the capital of chic and romance. But is that the real reason why we stand straight and walk tall, or is it the way we were brought up? Many of us were raised to stand and move in a way that denotes presence and class. I don't think that is necessarily innate; I think it can be learned.

Carole Bouquet embodies French class. It has often been said that Carole Bouquet "was a cold beauty." I had the chance to see her recently and can confirm she is a dazzlingly gorgeous sixty year old, with keen eyes and a firm figure, who was anything but cold. Nonstop smiles and beguiling allure. A magnificent lesson for women everywhere.

Crêpes

The Parisian woman is "slender" but a gourmand who loves crêpes! To calm her hunger pangs between appointments, regain strength after a session of Pilates, get over a setback, or enjoy a welcome treat in the middle of a long afternoon of shopping, the Parisian will, without guilt, treat herself to a "small" crêpe with lemon or apricot jam and then eat only a simple vegetable soup for dinner. At home, she will be content to make a nice stack of wheat crêpes for her children, while at the *crêperie* she dives into a buckwheat crêpe stuffed with ham and grated cheese, followed by a nice dessert crêpe. Accompanied of course by a glass of cider. You should know that there are two types of crêpes in Paris: one from a *crêperie*, the legendary Breton specialty, served at the table as a dish to eat with knife and fork; and the other "to go" that you buy from street vendors or the counters outside a café or brasserie. The Parisian specialty par excellence, "to go" crêpes, eaten standing, are prepared to order and served in plastic wrap. How to recognize a good crêpe? The dough of a crêpe "to be eaten at the table" must be thin and its filling must be fresh and homemade so you can eat several. While a "to go" crêpe that is eaten standing must be rich and nutritious, given that you are going to eat only one! The dough must be thicker to hold up well without dripping on your blouse. Eating one requires practice to avoid a whipped-cream mustache or a big chocolate stain, which is nice but not really a sign of Parisian elegance and glamour. Crêpes *flambée* with Grand Marnier should be served hot and still flaming! Tradition requires that they be served with a scoop of vanilla ice cream. Note that the French crêpe is prepared without yeast, unlike American pancakes or Russian blintzes.

HISTORY
At the end of the nineteenth century, the Paris-Brest railway was inaugurated, and thousands of Bretons arrived at the Gare Montparnasse to seek their fortune in Paris. That is still the area with the best crêperies in town. My favorite one is *Les Cormorans*.

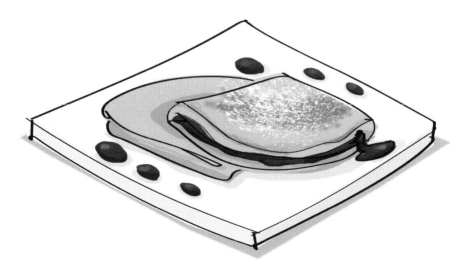

Croissant

LINKS
- Baguette
- Perfume
- Supermarket

The aroma of a croissant fresh from the oven is a characteristic scent of Paris. Especially in the morning, even though it is increasingly eaten at any time of day, the croissant is the basic Parisian breakfast par excellence, eaten in a hurry while drinking coffee (at the counter), on the street at the entrance of a bakery, or at the office while your computer is booting up. It's a good way to start the day.

Due to the Parisian woman's increasing distrust of everything industrial, there is a new generation of pastry chefs in Paris. With quality products and traditional methods, they are stimulating consumers to

HISTORY
It is said that Marie Antoinette imported the croissant from Vienna about 1780 and that they were first made in Paris in a bakery on the Rue Dauphine. The recipe was described in 1906 in *Auguste Colombié*'s culinary encyclopedia, where they are called "bakery croissants" and are described as a light puff pastry.

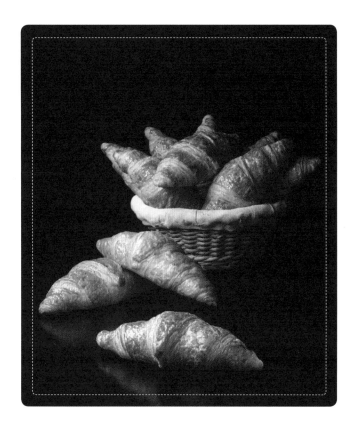

MY TIP
How to recognize a butter croissant? Generally, croissants made with vegetable fat take the form of a crescent while a butter croissant has a longer shape. However, bakeries that make only butter croissants prefer the half-moon shape. If in doubt, don't hesitate to ask. Just between us, there's a little trick for identifying fresh, homemade croissants: in the pastry shop, ask if you can "freeze" the croissants you want to buy. If they are honest and their croissants are "industrial," they will tell you not to do it.

demand ever higher standards of quality. Beware of pastry chefs who offer croissants that are soft and flat, full of air, too greasy, or over-cooked and dry.

A "croissant tour" is a delightful way to discover Paris. Many neighborhood bakeries make delicious croissants, and it's up to you to judge the color, crispness, lightness, and quality of the ingredients. My favorites are those of *Gérard Mulot* in Saint-Germain-des-Prés—fabulous and just minutes from home. You need only smell them to recognize the exceptional quality—an indescribably crisp pastry with the authentic taste of pure butter and a golden brown crust. The croissants from *Paul* are also excellent (photo). The Ispahan croissant from *Pierre Hermé* is original yet very good.

Croque-monsieur

Although Marcel Proust's madeleine is known around the world, not many know that the *croque-monsieur* (a sort of toast with ham and grilled cheese) also had its moment of glory in the famous French writer's *In Search of Lost Time*. In fact, there is a passage that tells how the Marquise Madeleine de Villeparisis ordered "croque-monsieur and egg with cream." Since that time, the *croque-monsieur* has been elevated to a higher gastronomic rank, having been invented in 1910 in a café on the Boulevard des Capucines, to become a "classic" of Parisian brasseries today. In the early twentieth century Parisians seemed to appreciate

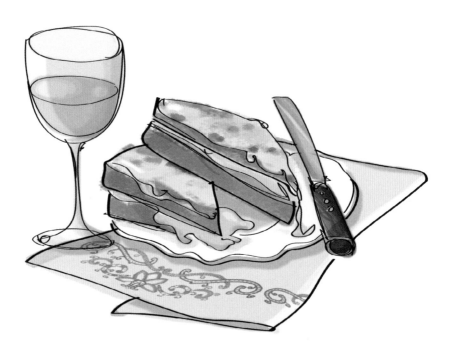

this strange sandwich consisting of slices of Swiss cheese and ham between two slices of buttered bread toasted in a mold. It is, in short, the ancestor of today's street food. Over the years, the *croque-monsieur* found itself mired in semi-industrial mediocrity, becoming a sort of sponge to be heated in the microwave. But later, with Italian sandwiches and bruschetta becoming fashionable, the *croque-monsieur* is once again very much appreciated, becoming the king of a Parisian woman's quick lunch. However, finding the right *croque-monsieur* in Paris is not easy: each of us has our own ideas about taste and nutrition and, when talking with my girlfriends, opinions on this matter are really divergent. If, lately, the fashion is a *croque-monsieur* made up of large slices of homemade bread like that of the *Poilâne* bakery, I literally go crazy for the ultra-classic of yore: splendid, full-bodied, and thick, made of quality sliced bread, crisp and golden-brown inside, a mountain of cheese, not too much *béchamel* sauce, and above all, quality cooked ham, all accompanied by a few leaves of green salad (a single variety) and a glass of white wine. I also go crazy for the *croque-madame*, a toast garnished with an egg that explodes and drips from the first forkful (yum!). Or for the *croque-monsieur* of the *Hôtel George V*—a pleasure to the nth degree, especially if accompanied by their legendary fries! However, the real star of the moment is the *croque-monsieur* of chef Yannick Alléno at the *Palais Brongniart*: two extra thin slices of bread, ham, and *béchamel* sauce mixed with *Comté* and Swiss cheese—low calory and so feminine! In any case, what really matters is that the *croque-monsieur* is crisp and soft at the same time and that it keeps its typical appearance of toast—that is, without becoming too elaborate a dish and overly rich with *béchamel* sauce, threatening to turn into a calorie bomb or a dish that makes you nauseous. For lovers of the *croque-monsieur* who can't decide which recipe is best for them, *La Maison du Croque-Monsieur* in Montparnasse offers many original *croque-monsieurs*. My absolute favorite is the vegetarian: goat cheese, sun-dried tomatoes, mushrooms, and walnuts. I just love chef Yves Camdeborde's *croque-monsieur* recipe. Chef Camdeborde's mini *croque-monsieurs* are heavenly with a glass of white wine at cocktail hour.

E

Eating Right

Parisian women are inundated with contradictory messages about diets from women's magazines. What's best? The Mediterranean diet? The high-protein, vegan, or neurotransmitter diet? One thing's for sure—today we know the point is not to be skinny, it's to be healthy. Today's Parisian women understand that good nutrition is the way to ward off a host of illnesses and to stay slim as well. Even if she can't resist a crunchy fresh baguette thickly coated with salty butter and luscious blueberry jam or fattening buttery croissants, she knows the importance

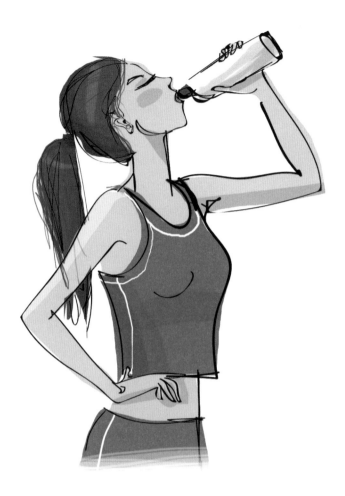

of a healthy lifestyle for the whole family and seeks to establish a balanced diet. She looks for fresh, natural products when she can and tries to buy less industrially processed foods. Of course, a busy life in a big city like Paris does not always make it easy to shop responsibly. When time permits, the Parisian loves buying fresh produce at farmers markets, but she'll put up with big grocery stores when there's no other choice.

Here are the rules that Hervé Grosgogeat, a nutritionist

and writer specialized in biology and sports medicine, teaches his patients in Paris:

"Most meals should consist of brightly colored foods; don't skip meals; eat three meals a day at rather precise times; avoid saturated fats; choose lean meats; eat more fiber; drink tea, preferably green tea; drink fresh-squeezed juices; drink a liter and a half of water a day; avoid processed foods like white flour and sugar; prefer whole wheat bread and avoid chemical yeast-based breads; if you can't do without sugar, use only natural substitutes; quit smoking; go out of town for some fresh air; avoid products based on phthalates and parabens; replace white rice with brown, basmati, or Thai rice with a lower glycemic index; give up sweets, industrial snacks, and sugary fruit drinks; remember to do at least thirty minutes of exercise per day; munch on raw fruit and vegetables with joy: celery, carrots, apples and pears, etc."

Elegance

People often talk about the elegance and "harmonious gracefulness" of Parisian women. But what's really behind this concept that has been the shared objective of all couture houses for centuries, the basic rule of French style? To what do we owe this reputation? Is it because we give the appearance of simple sophistication in our figures and movements? Or because we dress with simple refinement, secretly terrified of being classed as tasteless due to too much bling or artificial improvements? Our French education teaches us the ability to avoid excess; a sort of game of subtraction that helps us retain our essential chic. We learn from a very young age that, to be elegant, we have to dress in such a way that our elegance isn't visible to others and that "if we're too elegant, we stop being elegant," as my friend Manon told me yesterday. According to Voltaire: "Elegance comes from correctness and charm." So refinement and moderation are the

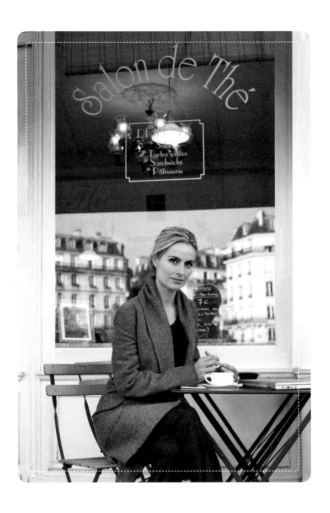

MY TIP

Here's what Professor Marramao has to say: "True elegance is not resolved in the superficial esthetics of an image narcissistically or spectacularly exhibited, but is expressed by the single detail, unique and not able to be copied, with which each of us enters into a relationship with others and with the outside world. Respecting the natural world and the human and non-human beings that surround us. Being able to convey strong emotions without being indiscreet. Demonstrating interest in the things that happen around us, holding high passion and tension toward others, preventing their degeneration into trivial curiosity. All this is elegance. But elegance also means avoiding showing your skills and talents. Elegance is the art of putting others at ease."

foundation of the Parisian woman's clothing style. According to the Italian philosopher Giacomo Marramao, whom I recently interviewed:

"France must surely owe its sobriety to the Republican revolution that shaped its personality and made execrable any display of wealth. Over the centuries, the French have learned the precious arts of nonchalance and irony as the expression of a deep-rooted self-awareness. Their sense of social belonging is less and less linked to image and increasingly recognizable in gestures and ways of behavior that reflect and, together, filter out one's inner life, leaving only a glimpse of the deepest emotional reactions."

The Parisian woman's elegance is expressed in the choice of accessories, moderate but effective, to complement her basic wardrobe.

• Don't put too much on when you're getting ready. The same applies for makeup—for an elegant Parisian look, make a choice: bright red lipstick or ultra-made-up eyes. The rule is moderation.

• Choose what you want to enhance. Your neck, your waist, your face, a gorgeous necklace, a low-cut dress, the cut of a jacket that looks great on you—but not all at once.

• Take care of your smile! It's good to get dressed up, but the best lipstick in the world won't look great when it shows off stained or chipped teeth, and the same applies for a mini-skirt and badly groomed legs. If you want to show off an asset, make sure beforehand that you're not going to draw attention to a fault! Whatever the case may be, the basic rule of elegance is "looking after our body."

• Check your social manners. Looking good with classy clothes isn't enough to give an elegant finale if the manners don't follow suit. Things you should stop right now: noisy gum chewing, unrefined gestures, coarse language, and a loud voice. A bit of self-criticism is the first step on the road to elegance.

"There's no elegance without inner elegance," said Yves Saint-Laurent. Spoken by a high-fashion giant, these words assume all their power in this modern materialistic world, often superficial and politicized. In theory, we all agree, but we need to remember it to fix it in our minds.

F

Factory Store

For the Parisian woman, the word *usine* (factory) does not evoke a Renault or Airbus assembly line but the outlet stores, *magasins d'usine*, with "factory" prices, where she can find her favorite clothing brands. Fabulous places where she can purchase luxury or vintage items at wholesale prices—in other words, without going broke.

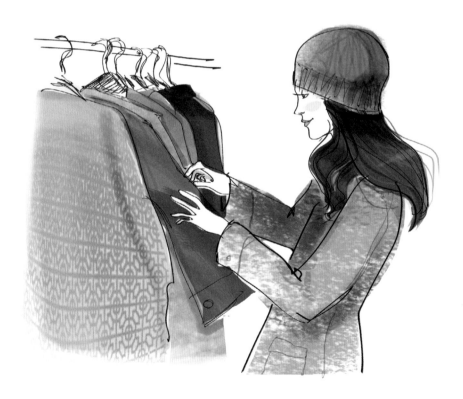

MY TIP
I found this website that lists the best outlets: *www.lesmagasinsdusine. com* (*Île de France* section). Be sure to check that the addresses are still current, as things change quickly in Paris!

In Paris, we don't like imitations, and even though, like many other women, our budget is limited, we love the quality of big-name designer products. So these stores are a godsend for us, especially if you are in the heart of Paris and don't want to travel twenty miles to buy a *Sonia Rykiel* sweater or *Repetto* ballerinas at reduced prices! We are always hunting for any new address that we discover through our fashionable friends. Because if Paris and its suburbs abound in particular stores, the difficulty lies in finding new places. My favorites: *Azzedine Alaia Stock Paris* in the 4th arrondissement and *A.P.C. Surplus* in the 18th.

Fashion Shopping

The Parisian woman does not follow the trends and dictates of the labels and catwalks but gives them only a distracted glance, because her way of shopping and filling her wardrobe is personal. She prefers to have a few beautiful but quality things—without disdaining quantity if the opportunity presents itself (sales of famous designer labels, private sales, or outlets). When not shopping online, during her lunch break, on sites like *Sézane* of my friend *Morgane Sézalory*, which are all the rage in Paris now, the Parisian woman shops in her district—either the Rive Gauche or the Rive Droite (Left Bank, Right Bank). This concept of the different banks of the Seine is fundamental to understand, not because they imply two very different ways of dressing, but because the two "genres" are rivals. However, the "Rive Gauche Parisian woman," who dotes on the eclectic shops of Saint-Germain-des-Prés, willingly crosses the Seine to visit the trendy boutiques and designers in the Marais, the special and chic ones of the Palais-Royal and the Boulevard Beaumarchais, or the luxury designers of the so-called Golden Triangle, where she buys the basic items of her wardrobe (trying to pay less). While the Parisian "yuppie" of the "Rive

LINKS
• Blue
• Sales
• Shoes
• Wardrobe

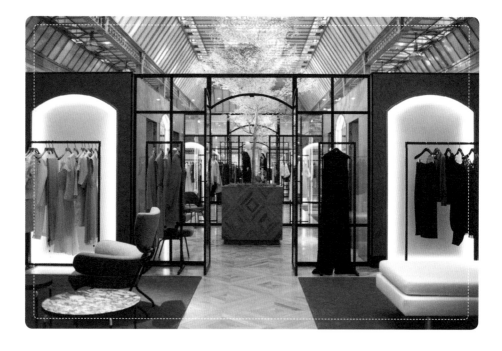

Gauche" is a *habitué* of shops in the Rue de Passy, the 17th arrondissement, the Avenue Montaigne, the Boulevard Haussmann, the Rue des Martyres, and Rue de Pigalle (the bohemian area in vogue), she does not disdain going to the Rive Gauche. So, it's a hypocritical borderline! Two things are certain: whether Rive Gauche or Rive Droite, the *Parisienne* knows what she wants and where to find it thanks to a well-maintained and updated address book. To each her own department store—for one *Galeries Lafayette* and *Printemps*; for the other *Le Bon Marché Rive Gauche*—is the place to be!

Rive Gauche (Left Bank)
In the heart of Paris, Saint-Germain-des-Prés, Sèvres Babylone, and Rue de Rennes are the not-to-be-missed places for Parisian shopping. The windows of the great designers compete and all the ready-to-wear brands are there. Just wander around calmly for three or four hours

and you've done the tour! Don't forget to stop for tea at *Ladurée* or for lunch at *Café de Flore* (but there's no lack of places). Rue Bonaparte is a must, and Rue des Quatre Vents, with its quirky shops, is not to be missed. Start your tour at the beginning of the Rue de Condé, continue along Rue Saint-Sulpice and Rue de Tournon, and finish in the Rue Guisarde, Rue des Canettes, Rue Madame, and Rue Jacob—in short, all the streets around Boulevard Saint-Germain. If you don't have enough time to see everything, take a general tour, then take Rue du Four to the *Bon Marché*, where you'll find all the top brands concentrated in one place. If you love shoes, Rue du Cherche Midi and Rue de Grenelle are the streets for you!

Rive Droite (Right Bank)
The gardens of the Palais-Royal, which are bordered by the Galleries of Montpensier and Valois, teem with artisans and prestigious and trendy brands that have chosen this district to showcase themselves to the world. Besides being beautiful, the district is essential for targeted shopping. Just a few minutes away are Place des Victoires and the Rue Saint-Honoré. Continue your tour toward the Marais. Here you can shop while strolling around Place des Vosges, Rue des Rosiers (a pedestrian mall), Rue des Francs-Bourgeois, and Rue du Temple. Absolutely not-to-be-missed, and with all the trendy brands. One of my favorites in the area is *Suite.341*, a trendy fashion concept store that houses the collections of *Maje*, *Sandro*, and *Claudie Pierlot*. A ten-minute walk away, the Boulevard Beaumarchais, also called "Haut Marais," is a must for shopping—very nice, with the famous *Merci* (also a concept store but for clothing, decorations, and food) and many big ready-to-wear labels that have set up here in recent years.
The district between Haussmann, Saint-Lazare, and l'Opéra is the commercial heart of Paris. It houses the famous department stores. The fantastic shop windows in the quarter are wonderful at Christmas! Rue Tronchet,

which connects Boulevard Haussmann to the Madeleine,
is particularly interesting. From there you can reach the
Rue Royale, Rue du Faubourg Saint-Honoré, and finally
Rue Saint-Honoré.
So-Pi (South of Pigalle) is the Parisian neighborhood
in vogue! This bohemian area is filled with vintage shops.
Rue des Martyrs, the main artery connecting the 9th
arrondissement and Montmartre, is the start of another
tour appreciated for its renowned "shopping stroll."
Not to be missed for lovers of jewelry and unusual
accessories is the boutique of designer *Emmanuelle
Zysman*. There are also many ready-to-wear brands:
Ba&sh, Kookai, Sandro, Maje, and *Les Petites*. Montmartre
is home to arty places like the *Spree* concept store
on Rue la Vieuville, which combines clothing, furniture,
design, and an art gallery.

Femininity

What do we mean when we speak of the Parisian woman's
femininity? I have asked dozens of people,
in France and abroad, and the replies focused mostly
on a combination of "elegance and sex appeal." They also
spoke of an enviable figure, which is the same thing. But
isn't Parisian femininity also a matter of attitude? A mix
of propriety and emancipation, associated with
a light gait, cultured language, and graceful gestures—and
perhaps a bit of lipstick or high heels as icing
on the cake? In reality, there are 1,001 ways to be feminine,
and the Parisian woman usually plays the card of a certain
disinterested class associated with a certain *je ne sais quoi*
(I don't know what) that comes from within, plus a warmth
and indecipherable iciness—a temperament that passes
in a moment from self-parody and scathing humor to
melancholy and fragility. Whether her femininity
is inherited from her mother or learned, the Parisian
seduces by creating relationships with others—and not

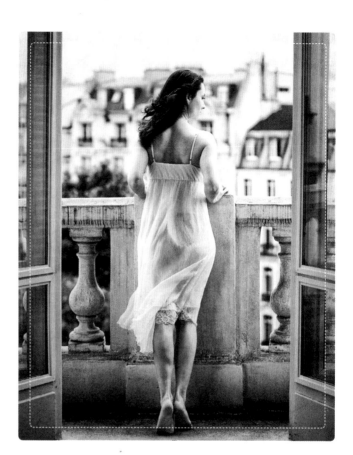

just in order to feel desirable in the eyes of men. In any case, judging from the surveys, being feminine, in Paris and elsewhere, is what most women say they want when using the services of image consultants. So, it is a topical subject even for Parisian women!

Flaws

Even if the *Parisienne* has become a marketing concept described in numerous works as a bit deliberately stereotyped, it is clear that one cannot generalize, neither with regard to her merits nor her minor flaws. Not all

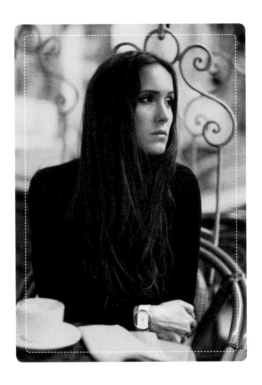

Parisian women are chic and slender, not all are in a hurry, and not all are difficult. The Parisian woman's defects can be read between the lines of this curious book, so I will not go on at length. In any case, here are some answers to the most common observations made about us:

• "The Parisian is always over the top."
Paris offers so much! So she must be a perfect woman who is talked about!
• "The Parisian is difficult."
She thinks in this way she shows independency ... Don't despair, over the next twenty years she will overcome this defect ...
• "The Parisian is cold."
On the second date, you will see that she is even more so. But after you have earned her trust, she is extremely sociable and friendly.

• "The Parisian is a snob."
Given that Paris is the capital of elegance, glamour, and culture, she has to prove to those who approach her that she is one of the fortunate who live here and knows the "best" of the city. You're right, that's no justification. But paradoxically she is open and curious when she lowers her shield of coldness.
• "The Parisian woman is never completely satisfied, is hypercritical, and is always right."
I don't know why. Education, competitiveness, or cultural tradition? I hope that Parisians will be lenient with the contents of this book. Even though, before writing, I interviewed a sampling of three hundred Parisian women of all ages, I never had the opportunity to ask an opinion in private …
• "The Parisian is stressed and in a hurry."
… like all women of the great capitals who fight against time for fear of being late and not being able to do everything.

Flowers

Maybe it's because she can no longer stand the grayness that the Parisian woman adores flowers. Or is it due to her natural inclination for romanticism and aesthetics? Whatever the reason, she has well-defined tastes, knows what she wants, and never chooses a bouquet in a hurry. Especially if it's for her! A perfectionist in touch with the depths of her soul, she arranges the flowers in her apartment or in her wedding bouquet in a way that gives her pleasure and evokes emotions, with their scent, their color, or their shape. Montaigne's phrase could be her motto: "If life is but a passage, in this passage let us, at least, sow flowers."
Every florist in the world will tell you—the French love white flowers! In the living room or the kitchen, sophisticated or simple wildflowers, white is the most

LINKS
• Avenue Montaigne
• Interiors
• Perfume

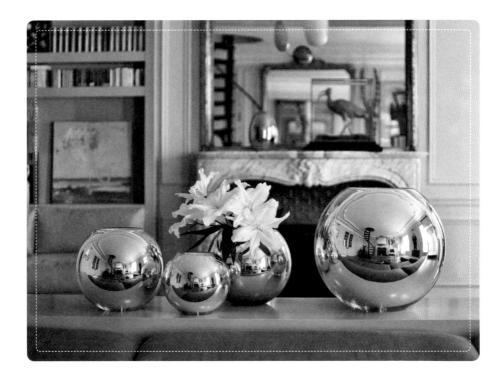

popular color: an always trendy gardenia, a classic bouquet of tulips, but even combinations such as roses and white hydrangeas, roses and agapanthus, or a beautiful bouquet of lilacs or peonies, depending on the season.

Those who love classic and very elegant bouquets buy from *Adriane M* (Rue Saint-Dominique) or *Stéphane Chapelle* (near the Comédie-Française), two of the best florists and gardeners of Paris. Master florist Stéphane Chapelle is a favorite among fashion houses and neighborhood residents. He is a genuine artist, whose compositions reflect both his Norman country soul and Parisian notions of luxury. Whatever he is called on to create, from a simple bouquet to complex scenography, his works are sober and natural. Don't you just adore trendy town & country style?

HISTORY
Did you know that Madame Prévost opened the first flower shop in the Palais-Royal in 1830? Let yourself be captivated by the beautiful flowers of the master florist of Rue du Faubourg Saint-Honoré, *Lachaume.* Just the idea that Marcel Proust used to come here every day to put a flower in his lapel fills us with emotion.

In Paris, those with a passion for orchids use *Sylvain George,* the great specialist of the capital. In his wonderful shop behind the Place des Victoires are various types of orchids (*phalaenopsis, odontoglossum, paphiopedilum, cattleya,* and *oncidium*), coexisting in very sophisticated arrangements.

The chic and trendy Parisian bohemian woman instead loves composing her own romantic country bouquets, buying flowers from *Monceau Fleurs* while riding around on her bicycle. This chain is a sort of flower supermarket, where customers can create their own bouquets of very good quality and price rate.

I particularly love the shop *Un peu, beaucoup.* François Lequesne is an authentic creator of environments and emotions, and his floral arrangements are actual stories told by protagonists of the plant kingdom.

Fond of tradition, the Parisian woman, paradoxically, also loves everything that is contemporary, cutting edge, or exclusive. Hence the success of the sumptuous flower arrangements of Jeff Leatham in the *Four Seasons George V.* You will find a breath of fresh air at *Odorantes,* a florist specializing in fragrant flowers. Nice, *n'est-ce pas?*

It is impossible to speak of the flowers of Paris without evoking the public gardens and their colorful flowerbeds, the Tuileries on the Rive Droite, and, on the Rive Gauche, the Jardin du Luxembourg and the Jardin des Plantes (the first public garden created in the capital). Then there's the flower market in the center of Paris and the scarlet flowers along the Avenue Montaigne and balconies filled with begonias, geraniums, and hydrangeas! Can we call Paris the "city of flowers"?

Special attention must be paid to the wedding bouquet. In the last few years, the Parisian woman's wedding bouquet has become less classic, made of roses picked in the garden, studded with sweet peas, and mixed peonies, wild plants, or even colored dahlias. It is much more "country romantic." White is the color most used, sometimes accented by ivory or pink. *Maison Vertumne* is one of the places not to be missed. More confidential and fashionable is *DeBeaulieu* for a wonderful retro bouquet. Today it is trendy to wear crowns of fresh flowers worn like a diadem in your hair, adorned with small silk roses or lace.

Foie Gras

The first thing to know about foie gras is never to call it *pâté* in front of a Parisian. It ain't chopped liver! *Parisiennes* take foie gras very seriously. It is part of our culinary heritage. Pâté, at best, is a poor cousin of foie gras, and confusing the two is tantamount to sacrilege. It would be like saying that pheasant under glass is "just chicken" or that caviar is "just fish eggs." Foie gras is fatted goose or duck liver. Whether it comes from a gourmet caterer or the supermarket, whether we truthfully enjoy the taste or not, foie gras is sacred! So even if you think it looks like liverwurst, call it by its rightful name. If you're a guest at a Parisian home, simply tell your hostess *votre foie gras est délicieux* (your foie gras is delicious)—that's enough!

Foie gras is sold fresh, *mi-cuit* (half cooked), or *cuit* (cooked). It can be served hot, lightly pan-fried, for example. Or it might be presented cold in terrine form,

LINKS
• Gastronomy
• Silverware
• Wine

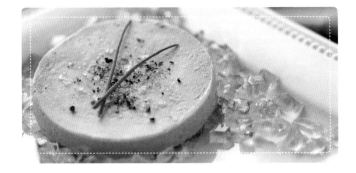

and cut into thin slices directly in your plate. Foie gras is sometimes also served on a bed of gelatin straws. Like most *Parisiennes*, I prefer quality foie gras and bread, simply and elegantly served, to cheap foie gras with a flashy presentation. If you serve your foie gras on a plate, use a serving fork and spoon.

How does one eat foie gras elegantly and according to the rules of French tradition? In Paris, where foie gras is a luxury, it must be served with a befitting ritual. For example, only hot, pan-fried foie gras can be eaten with a knife and fork. Otherwise, only a fork is used, never a knife. Don't even touch your knife, even if your hostess or the waiter has set one by your plate. Why? Because this would be kind of impoliteness towards your hostess, as if to say: "Your foie gras is so tough it needs a knife to be cut."

THE RECIPE
A real Parisian woman knows how to make homemade foie gras. I suggest an easy method and one that makes a good impression: buy readymade foie gras and serve it "Parisian-style." Here's one way that's easy and tasty.

Sautéed Foie Gras

Serves 4
4 slices of duck or goose liver foie gras, 1/3 cup each
4 slices of bread thickly cut
4 apples (for cooking)
3 1/2 tbsp. butter
1/2 beet and a whole endive
salt, pepper

Toast the slices of bread and then cut them into rounds. Peel the apples, cut them up into thick slices, and sauté in a skillet with butter until golden. Set aside. Place the slices of foie gras in the freezer for 5 minutes.

Meanwhile, clean the skillet, warm it up and arrange the slices of foie gras (without fat) in it, cooking each side for 1 minute. Remove and place on a paper towel.

Place the toasted bread rounds in a baking dish and top with the apple slices, a pinch of sea salt, and some pepper.

Before serving, place the baking dish in a pre-heated oven (400°F) for 3 minutes.

Serve the slices of toast accompanied by a beet and endive salad (julienne the vegetables). Drizzle with hazelnut oil and Xeres vinegar.

So why do you sometimes see foie gras spread on toast at supposedly high-class receptions? To make it easier to serve, would be my guess. Or perhaps they have forsaken traditional Parisian *savoir-vivre*.

French Kiss

Few places are more romantic than Paris. What other city has so many magical spots for a passionate kiss? Do you know the Vert-Galant square on the Île de la Cité—the very heart of Paris, where the light flickers with romantic hues and the neighboring monuments seem to dance in rhythm

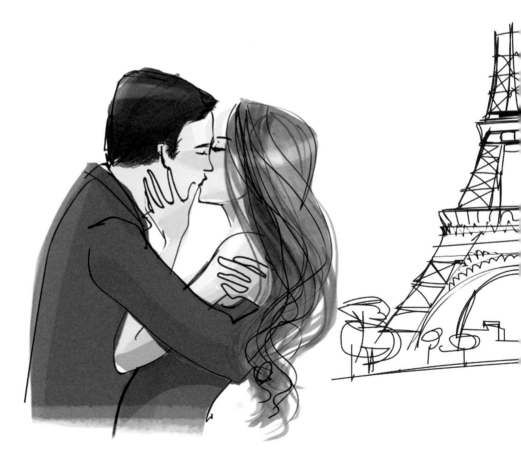

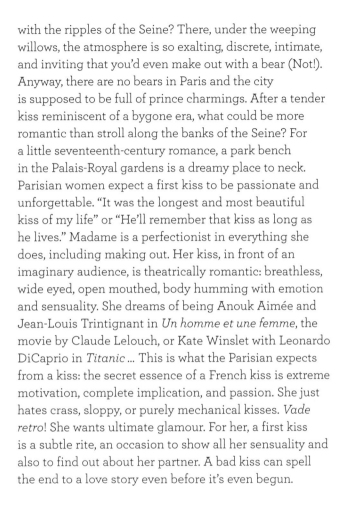

with the ripples of the Seine? There, under the weeping willows, the atmosphere is so exalting, discrete, intimate, and inviting that you'd even make out with a bear (Not!). Anyway, there are no bears in Paris and the city is supposed to be full of prince charmings. After a tender kiss reminiscent of a bygone era, what could be more romantic than stroll along the banks of the Seine? For a little seventeenth-century romance, a park bench in the Palais-Royal gardens is a dreamy place to neck. Parisian women expect a first kiss to be passionate and unforgettable. "It was the longest and most beautiful kiss of my life" or "He'll remember that kiss as long as he lives." Madame is a perfectionist in everything she does, including making out. Her kiss, in front of an imaginary audience, is theatrically romantic: breathless, wide eyed, open mouthed, body humming with emotion and sensuality. She dreams of being Anouk Aimée and Jean-Louis Trintignant in *Un homme et une femme*, the movie by Claude Lelouch, or Kate Winslet with Leonardo DiCaprio in *Titanic* ... This is what the Parisian expects from a kiss: the secret essence of a French kiss is extreme motivation, complete implication, and passion. She just hates crass, sloppy, or purely mechanical kisses. *Vade retro*! She wants ultimate glamour. For her, a first kiss is a subtle rite, an occasion to show all her sensuality and also to find out about her partner. A bad kiss can spell the end to a love story even before it's even begun.

Friendship

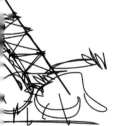

Friendship is an important feeling for a Parisian woman and, along with family and education, is one of the pillars of her equilibrium. Cold and distant at first, she gradually lets herself go, becoming accessible, open, and friendly if she likes you and feels that there is the potential for a sincere and lasting friendship. If she finds you to her liking, she will not hesitate to suggest going for a drink

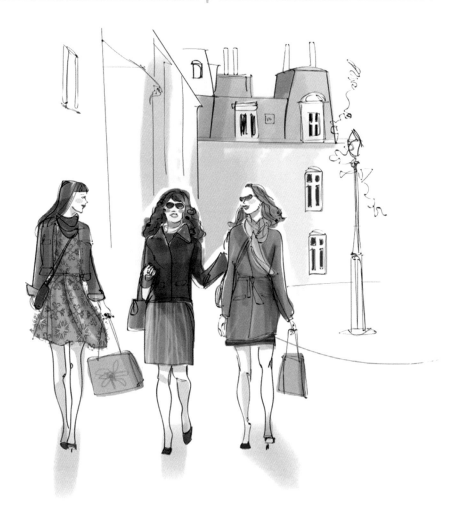

to chat and get to know each other or invite you to lunch to join the circle of her best friends. Like an adolescent, she will open her heart to those who convey trust or at least sympathy. Moreover, her well-being owes much to the presence of her friends.

In Paris, like everywhere else in the world, the important thing is regular contact to exchange impressions and the latest little secrets. The Parisian woman sees friendship as

The Parisian woman enjoys gathering her friends around a delicious dish of homemade food. One recipe that's particularly convivial is Bœuf Bourguignon, a dish that's ideal for someone who has a day job because it can be made in advance. And it's even more delicious when it's reheated the next day.

Bœuf Bourguignon

Serves 6

2 lb. 3 oz. beef rump cut up into squares about 2 in. per side
1 1/2 tbsp. oil
2 tbsp. flour for the roux
1 cup light cooking liquid or stock, the wine from the marinade
2 tbsp. chopped mushrooms
1/2 bouquet garni
1/2 clove of garlic
For the marinade
1 3/4 cup fine red wine
1/2 medium-sized onion finely chopped
1/4 bay leaf
2 stalks of parsley
1/2 sprig of thyme
1 tbsp. extra-virgin olive oil
salt, pepper
Side dish
4 1/2 oz. lean bacon
12 small onions
1/2 cup mushrooms
3 1/3 tbsp. butter

Mix all the ingredients of the marinade and dip the meat into the mixture, for a richer flavor. Leave in the marinade for a few hours. Wash and clean the mushrooms. Chop the stems into two-three pieces and the caps into two-four pieces. Sauté over high heat in 2 tablespoons of butter. Drain and set aside.

Remove the rind from the bacon and dice into squares 1/2 inch per side. Place in a small skillet with cold water and cook for 5 minutes after the water starts boiling. Use a paper towel to pat the bacon dices dry. Heat 2 tablespoons of butter in the skillet you're going to use for the beef and brown the bacon over high heat together with the peeled, chopped onions. Remove from heat and combine with the side dish.

In the same fat, brown the pieces of meat after carefully patting them dry. Drain the fat from the skillet. Sprinkle the beef with flour and cook over very low heat stirring with a wooden spoon. Add the stock and the wine from the marinade, the chopped mushrooms, the bouquet garni, and the clove of garlic, mixing thoroughly. Bring to a boil. Cover and cook for 2 hours over low heat. Deglaze the sauce, which should be about 1/2 the original amount. Cover and continue to cook for another 30 minutes. Serve.

an opportunity to share authentic moments with another person, chatting, discussing more serious topics or heavy subjects, talking about everything and nothing, but freely without fear of being judged or betrayed. And yes, in this as well, the Parisian is demanding and gives her all.

Her best friend is always at her side, mentally or physically. The *Parisiennes*'s best friends are sincere and affectionate, promising to be available to each other at any time of the day or night, but without taking advantage. The Parisian would not hesitate to cancel an appointment with the President of the Republic to cheer up a girlfriend in need of her. A meeting is followed by a series of text messages or e-mails to keep updated. They have already talked about and experienced so many things together that there is no need to start from scratch each time. But beware, a secret is a secret, and if the best friend reveals confidential information to someone else, it's the end! No mercy. She wants truth, integrity, and reliability— without, however, demanding exclusivity like a teenager. Moreover, she knows how to surround herself with an ultra-sophisticated social network. There is a best male friend and girlfriends for going out to have fun, for culture, the gym, the child's school, and so on. There are friends for going shopping and those who like eating out and trying a new bistro or preparing lunch at home with friends.

I was explaining to Jenny, my friend from Philadelphia, that, in Paris, friends of friends are not necessarily our friends. The Parisian is a free woman who likes to choose her friends directly. But that doesn't prevent her from being kinder to them than strangers!

G

Galette des Rois

Who's going under the table? No, it's not a new Parisian game but the celebration of Epiphany. Every year on January 6 the ritual of the *galette des Rois* is performed with a crusty pastry pie filled with frangipane. It is

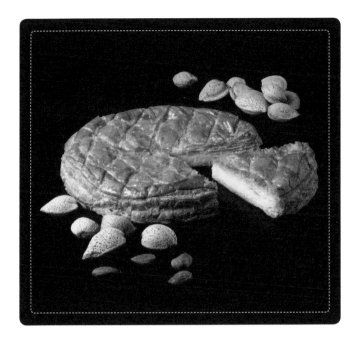

a tradition that lasts several days, to the great delight of our children, who all dream of the same thing: being the one who gets the *fève* (fava bean) and wears the golden crown. According to tradition, the *fève*, generally ceramic, is hidden inside the *galette*. The person who gets it is the king (or queen) for the day and gets to wear the crown. A gold paper crown! It's generally the youngest child who hides under the table and decides who gets which piece, called out by the person cutting the *galette:*
"Who's this piece for?"
"Justine."
"And this one?"
"Kevin."

... And so on. Impartiality in how the portions are served is guaranteed. As dentists know, it's also the day that most French people break a tooth! My favorite place for a gluten-free *galette des Rois* is *Sitron* (15 Rue Marie Stuart, 2nd arrondissement), for a classic *galette*, *Paul* (photo).

LINKS
• Baguette
• Bistro
• Eating Right
• Supermarket

Gastronomy

The Parisian woman's heart is balanced between the specialties of her home region (she is not necessarily born in Paris), international recipes, and fusion cuisine, not to mention the creations of Parisian master chefs. Like many of us, my friends Françoise and Julie are big fans of Gagnaire (if you're part of the in-crowd, you don't call him Chef Pierre Gagnaire). Nicole and Marion swear by Chef Yannick Alléno (who happens to be handsome). Personally, I'm fond of Chef Jean François Piège, whom I find simply wonderful, and also of Yves Camdeborde. I find him incredibly modern and simple.

Even though the Parisian loves world cuisine and yakitori, sushi, egg rolls, linguini, and panna cotta may be among

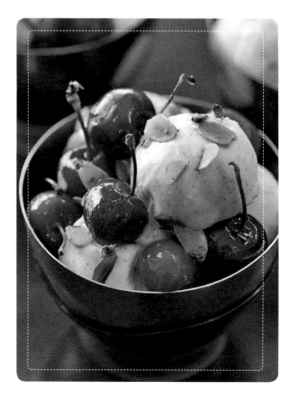

MY TIP
As it is in neighboring Italy, another land with excellent regional ingredients, French homestyle cooking has a lot of delicious traditional local recipes that are largely unknown abroad. Visit a Parisian brasserie or bistro, and if you're not in the mood for *boeuf bourguignon,* beef stew, or *choucroute alsacienne* (sauerkraut), ask what the products of the season are and try the simplest version.

her staple foods, she'll go absolutely ballistic, to say the least, if anyone dares criticize her French gastronomy, recognized by UNESCO as part of the "immaterial world's cultural heritage!" Tell us that French cuisine is too heavy, that there's too much sauce, or that a product is too bland, and see what happens. When it comes to French gastronomy, we mean business. Keeping that in mind, we hope you'll be open to all the dining experiences the *Parisienne* enjoys, including family recipes, gourmet foods, fusion, avant-garde molecular, and many others. As for typically French food, I'd say there are two main categories: gastronomic cuisine and home cooking.

• Gastronomic cuisine is like a symphony. Whereas in music, the maestro blends the sounds of a multitude of instruments into a sophisticated feast for the ears, so a master chef skillfully combines a variety of fresh ingredients into a symphony for your eyes, nose, and taste buds. Top-quality ingredients are only the starting point. The great chefs are true artists, and what really counts is the unique way their creative recipes subtly appeal to our senses. Are these examples of works by Pierre Gagnaire music to our ears? "Fondant of goose foie gras; slivers of lacquered pigeon; shallot, rubinette apple, and cinnamon marmalade; tamarillo pulp; and red kuri squash creamed with coconut milk."

At his flagship restaurant *Daniel* in New York, Chef Daniel Boulud showed that you could serve fine French cuisine outside France, using local products of high quality. This is possible when the chef, like a conductor who gets the most out of his musicians, makes the most of the products at his disposal to produce masterpieces such as "Four Story Hill farm-fresh squab: roasted breast meat with winter black truffle, foie-gras-stuffed legs, spelt wheat risotto, sauce flavored with truffle juice and twelve-year-old Dalmore scotch."

• Home cooking and good French ingredients are like chamber music. We use fewer ingredients so that their respective flavors really come through. In France we have

Pompadour Potato Tartiflette

Serves 4

2 lb. 3 oz. Pompadour potatoes
1 Reblochon cheese
1 tbsp. oil
5 oz. bacon
3 onions
1/2 cup heavy cream
1 pat of butter
salt and pepper

THE RECIPE
The Parisian woman loves to eat and loves comfort food. In the winter, to ward off the cold, between a detox smoothie and a healthy salad, she dares every now and then to cook a delicious tartiflette for her family and friends. Here's a traditional winter recipe, to be savored before a crackling fireplace...

Pre-heat the oven to 410°F. Boil the potatoes for about 15 minutes. Let cool, then cut into slices. Chop the onions then sauté in a skillet with some oil. Add the bacon and cook everything for about 10 minutes over medium heat. Butter a glass baking dish then add a layer of potatoes. Add the bacon and onions mixture. Sprinkle with pepper. Pour the cream over everything and then top with slices of Reblochon cheese. Bake for about 10 minutes. Potato tartiflettes must be prepared with quality potatoes, and I use Pompadour's, a *Label Rouge* French trademark, but you can use any kind of potatoes, just remember they have to be high quality.

a number of outstanding regional products the quality of which is backed by strict certification labels (for example, *AOC* or *Label Rouge*): Brittany artichokes, Prés Salé lambs, Limousin apples, Mont Saint-Michel Bouchot mussels, Grenoble walnuts, Loiret Gariguette strawberries, and Bresse poultry, to name just a few. Let's take a simple recipe made with Orleans asparagus, harvested before they emerge from the soil. A light *mousseline* sauce is used so as not to overwhelm their delicate flavor. Likewise, Brittany artichokes are best appreciated with a simple vinaigrette; anything fancier would overpower the taste. For something different, try a Noirmoutier Bonnotte (variety of small and very exclusive potato) topped by an Arcachon oyster—just fantastic—or some little gray Morbihan shrimps on a thin slice of a buttered French baguette, Collioure anchovy quiche, or Picardie Pompadour potatoes with Reblochon cheese sauce that shall exalt the aromas.

Grandma

Do you know what a *Parisienne* does when she receives roses? She recalls what her grandmother taught her: drop an aspirin into the water and they will keep longer. For a *Parisienne*, grandmothers are the greatest database of wisdom. What Frenchwoman can ever forget the wonderful vacations we spent with our grandmothers? Often, the kids spend August with their parents in Brittany or the southwest, two of the standard places for Parisian middle-class families. But July is a problem for mom and dad, who are working and/or have a million

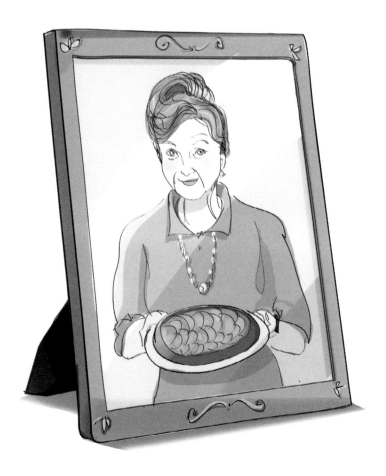

and one things to do. The kids take courses, go to summer or scout camp, but they can also spend some of July at one of their grandmas' family properties. And yay, at last! Some time off for the parents! Bonne-Maman, Mamie, Mamine, Moune, Mamina, Mima, Mouchka— whether we call them by an old fashioned nickname or a trendy new one, our grandmothers remain dear to our hearts and a pillar of our upbringing. In addition to creating her own album of memories, we add more material to our book of "grandma's" secrets and recipes. Rinsing your hair with a bit of chamomile, using leftover pastry to make little biscuits for tea, using yesterday's newspaper to clean the windows, putting an apricot stone in the jam, and stopping a soufflé from collapsing when you bring it to the table are among the many secrets of life! Thank you Grammie and Bonne Maman!

Gratin

It is well known that the best part of *au gratin* dishes is often the crust! In the kitchen, it is the upper part of a dish that is toasted during the final minutes of cooking to obtain a golden brown crust. The concept is so ancient and well known that Parisians have made it a popular

MY TIP
To enhance the crust or make it better or more consistent, sprinkle the dish you want to brown with grated cheese, breadcrumbs, or even toasted *pain d'épices* (bread with spices).

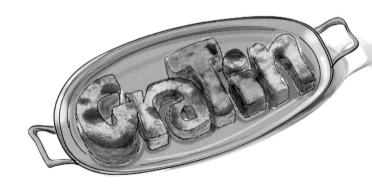

expression, "the gratin," meaning "the best," which, by analogy, became "the worldly elite, good people, high and good society, the aristocracy, the crème de la crème."
"Were you at the *Fiac* opening?"
"Yes, there was all the 'gratin' of Paris!"
To return to our delicious gratin, the French adore it, and it is often prepared as a main dish at home, especially in large families, because it is practical and comprehensive. Zucchini *au gratin,* leeks *au gratin,* and onion soup *au gratin*—to each her own recipe.

Endives and Ham *au gratin*

Serves 2
2 endives
2 slices of ham or Bresaola (lighter)
1 3/4 tbsp. butter
1/4 onion, cut into rings
1/2 lemon
salt and pepper
For the Mornay sauce
2 tbsp. flour
1 tbsp. butter
1 cup milk
2 oz. Gruyere cheese
salt, pepper, and nutmeg

THE RECIPE
This dish reminds me of my childhood. But I enrich this classic recipe with a personal touch: before placing the dish in the oven, I add two tablespoons of honey to maintain a slightly sweet flavor that offsets the bitterness of the endive.

Remove withered endive leaves. With a sharp knife, dig out and remove the inside of the stalk. Wash the endives with plenty of water and dry them immediately. Melt a teaspoon of butter in a saucepan. Add the onion and the endive. Sprinkle lemon juice so the endive will not oxidize. Add salt and pepper, cover, and simmer for one hour. Stir occasionally during cooking.

For the Mornay sauce: over medium heat, stir the flour with the butter. Let it barely cook. Pour in the cold milk all at once. Mix and bring to a boil. Add salt, pepper, and nutmeg and cook for five minutes. Away from the heat, add the grated cheese.

Cover each endive with half a slice of thin-cut ham or Bresaola. Place in a rectangular roasting pan and cover with Mornay sauce. Add lumps of butter and brown for five minutes at the top of a hot oven or, even better, on a grill.

Grayness

Did you know that a gray environment stimulates curiosity, reflection, and imagination? Can this be why Paris is so gray? With the sky, the mood, and the wardrobe, there is gray everywhere. Every year, they say that it is "the sovereign basic color of the fall wardrobe." The timeless shades of gray return relentlessly. The underground returns to the surface. Less rigorous than black, less flat and bright than white, gray allows us to pass a mild, neutral winter. So they say. The reference collections: *Acne Studio, Balenciaga, Chloé, Les Petites, Paul & Joe.* The latest trend of the moment is to wear even your hair gray (a bright, silvery, not discolored gray). I don't go along with it. I am more cheerful and wait impatiently for

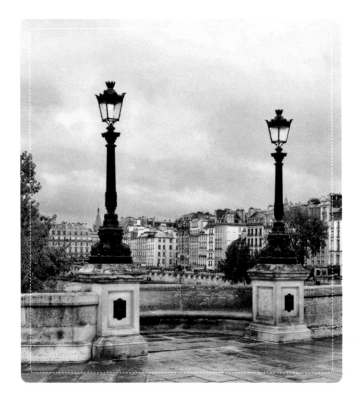

the first ray of sunlight that will make me forget the Parisian grayness for some hours or days! Even the pigeons never go out without their gray trench coats. But whether *Ramier* (ringdoves) or *Biset* (wild pigeons), our two local species, their uniform does not stop them from safely walking the streets of Paris in search of food.

While all *Parisiennes* dream of holidays in the sun, away from the grayness, it seems that the tourists are so dazzled by the beauty of Paris that they do not care about it. They see everything in color! You should note, however, that our weather is often capricious. The morning can begin gray and damp while, in the afternoon, a bright sun can appear to warm the hearts of Parisian women and give the city a sublime appearance, worthy of its reputation as the *Ville Lumière* (City of Light)!

H

Hair

Like her wit and her sense of humor, a Parisian woman's hair is one of her weapons of mass seduction. Whether it's because of her temperament or her upbringing, the Parisian likes to highlight her best features, especially her hair, her figure, and her smile. She enjoys taking care of her hair and is willing to spend a small fortune on masks, creams, and vinegars to make it healthy and shiny. She goes for a natural look, nothing that looks fake or sprayed into place. She wants a gentle breezy movement, not "holding power." Her hair should be well styled yet tousled for a smart casual look. Forget about weirdo looks, bizarre hair accessories, or pink streaks and tips. Hair color must be as natural as possible. A very discrete *balayage* with girlish golden highlights does it every time, and don't we know it! Admit it, my dear girlfriends: who hasn't gone into a hair salon brandishing a photo of herself as a girl and saying, "Can you give me highlights just like that?" Ponytails are still all the rage in Paris. So do all Parisian

LINKS
• Age
• Elegance
• Femininity
• Grayness

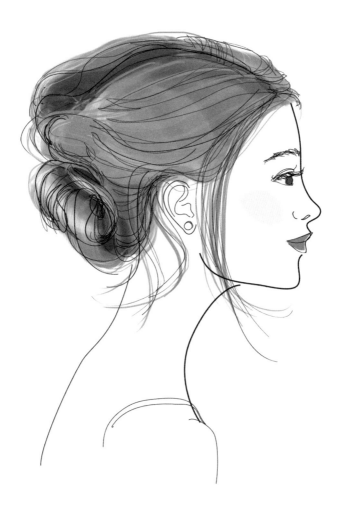

MY TIP
Take a look at women's hairstyles in ads for French luxury products (for example, *Aigle, Longchamp, Hermès, Louis Vuitton, Zadig & Voltaire, Lancel*). You'll notice long or shoulder-length hair—thick silky manes in movement. Take a good look at these hairstyles and see if you can copy them. And don't forget the rules above! If you're aiming for a Parisian look, it's best not to go out with a scrunchie in your hair. Instead opt for hairpins in an elegant but nonchalantly mussed chignon (bun), hide an elastic band with a strand of hair, or wear a pretty barrette. Personally, I like *Alexandre de Paris* "tortoise shell"–type barrettes. They come in black or colors. Pure class! They add a touch of elegance, and it's easy to let just a few locks of hair slip out for a deliberately "mussed" look.

dudes dig the "good girl" look that ponytails are supposed to portray? Surveys say yes, as long as it's occasional—not the woman's everyday style.

Don't blow-dry your hair too much. It dries out your hair, and who wants to look like an over-brushed Barbie doll! The Parisian prefers to let her hair dry naturally, the old-fashioned way—with a towel.

Heels

Have you heard a rumor that low heels will soon outdo stiletto heels in Paris? That four-inch heels are on their way out? Nonsense! The *Parisienne* may occasionally yearn for simpler and more comfy footwear and have trouble choosing between a lower and a higher heel,

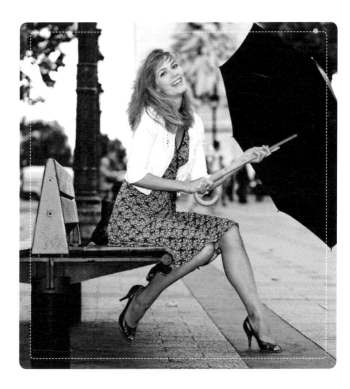

HISTORY
In the old days, when people said "high heels" they meant three inches. But for the last few seasons, some heel wearers have been getting carried away. Six inches are no longer just for the red carpet or the catwalk. You see *Parisiennes* in the square with their kids practically wearing stilts! Isn't there such a thing as too much? Heels are pretty if you wear them well, but thinking that real women can stroll along gracefully on heels half a foot high is science fiction!

but no way are we going to switch to one-inch heels for good! It is true that fashion magazines these days are trying to convince the masses that flats are feminine and glamorous, but I seriously doubt the Parisian woman will give up high heels any time soon. After all, she didn't spend a good eighteen years of her life learning to perch on four inches for nothing! She'll buy new flats for her wardrobe but remain faithful to her heels. Flats are more to slip into a bag "just in case." Our street interview shows the thoughts of women in Paris:

"Long hair and high heels—the essence of my femininity."
Clotilde, Rue Marbeuf, January 10
"My heels make me feel strong. They give me bearing and presence when I walk. Without them I'd feel like I was limping."
Lola, Place Vendôme, March 12
"I need heels to elongate my figure, otherwise I feel fat."
Laetitia, Rue de Rivoli, March 15
"I hate feeling short."
Romane, Rue de Passy, March 15
"I can stand tall before my business contacts."
Maëlys, Place de l'Opéra, February 12
"My back aches if wear flats, and I get cramps in my calves."
Charlotte, Rue du Louvre, March 16

How does a Parisienne choose the right heels?
• She tries on lots and lots—and not just the most expensive brands. There's more to life than *Academy, Acne, Dior, Roger Vivier, Louboutin*, and *Saint-Laurent*!
• She selects the right size, neither too small (scrunched up toes hurt) nor too big (if her foot slides around in the shoe, she'll walk funny, which is not exactly chic).
• Better a good three inches than a bad five inches. If the arch is comfortable and the foot is placed naturally, they're a pleasure to walk in; otherwise they can be a real nightmare.

MY TIP
If you're not used
to really high heels,
practice first. Your steps
should be closer and a
little slower than usual.
Be careful if you're
walking down stairs.
Imagining that there
are one hundred
photographers awaiting
you at the bottom of
the red carpet stairway
at the Cannes Film
Festival will give you
a little more grace. If
you can't walk naturally
in super-high heels,
then downsize. If your
feet are naturally
arched and your ankles
are well supported,
you'll walk more
naturally and sensually.

How does a Parisienne choose low heels?
• Whether she's selecting ballerinas, oxfords, boots,
or even sneakers, the Parisian woman is not simply
choosing footwear—she's considering how these shoes
will contribute to her overall look. Low is not necessarily
better or worse than high, it all depends.
• If you're used to wearing high heels, opt for the most
feminine pair of low heels in the store, the ones that will
make your legs look great and give you a sexy walk. Your
style may be athletic or businesslike, but you can still be
feminine and chic.
• Avoid fat thick soles; they weight down your ankle and
give you a masculine "hiker" look that is not appreciated
by guys and is often the butt of jokes among gals, like,
"are those orthopedic shoes you're wearing?"

Herbal Teas

After dinner is a delicate time when the Parisian woman
coddles her guests with a good ending that will leave them
with unforgettable memories of the evening. Comforting,
well-selected drinks and sweets are the essential rules of
the after-dinner art. And don't forget the relaxing herbal
teas that have surpassed even the best liqueurs! Even men
have begun to appreciate them. Boiling water and plants
makes a good combination—all the major brands of herbal
teas have identified a virgin market and have let their
imaginations run wild, creating infusions that guarantee
a good night's sleep. In short, everyone has her own recipe
for sweet dreams!
"Nature is always right. The positive effect that herbs have
on the treatment of common illnesses such as stress
or for liver or digestive problems is well known," says
my friend Marc Messegué, the famous phytotherapist
and herbalist.
Opt for an entertaining presentation on the tray. Be sure
to prepare it before the guests arrive because, when you

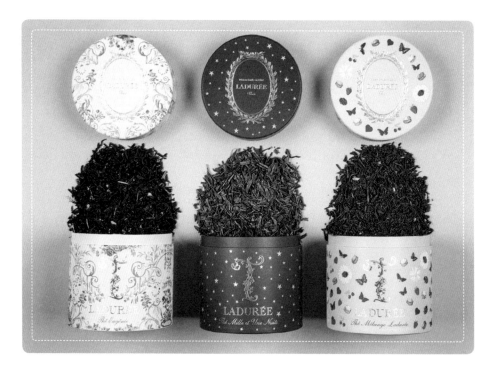

MY TIP
Offer your guests an assortment of herbal teas: linden and chamomile promote sleep; fennel, mint, and sage help the digestion; marjoram and verbena are relaxants; and green tea is a stimulant. A tea that's really trending in Paris right now is *1001 Nuits* by Ladurée, a Chinese green tea, both mild and spicy. A blend of rose, orange blossom, and ginger.

are sleepy, there's nothing more exasperating than waiting twenty minutes to be served some herbal tea. And, above all, at the end of dinner, don't run to fill the dishwasher, leaving your guests alone too long.

Verbena Liquor
If you want to satisfy fans of both of liqueurs and verbena, you can offer your guests an alternative herbal tea, made with your own hands:

Ingredients
• Verbena leaves
• Brandy (50% alcohol by volume)
• Sugar
• Water

After steeping for two months in the dark, filter: your homemade verbena liqueur is ready!

High Standards

If I had to sum up Parisian mentality, "high standards" would probably be it. We Parisians are too damned demanding. It's an attitude that's drummed into us at a tender age. You simply "must" get into the "right" daycare center and then into the "right" schools. If you're a "proper" young lady, you go to a debutante ball.

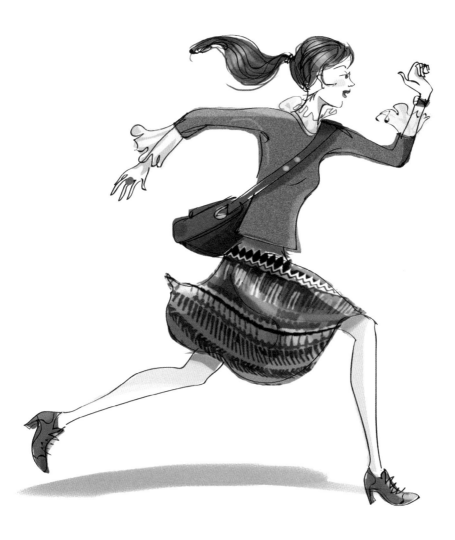

You choose the right career path and the right mate.
If you enter a marathon, you run to win.
There's no place for losers. I often tell my foreign friends,
"Parisians demand a lot of themselves and others, that's
why they're so stressed out all the time." Once
you've learned how to keep your standards high, the next
stage in life is to make all this look effortless.
You must never let on how hard it is for you to stay svelte,
stylish, and cultivated. And please never complain
or deplore. It has to appear natural! If only people knew
how many years of hard work it took to develop this
picture-perfect persona!
It is your role to embody flawless Parisian *savoir-vivre*.
The reputation of our glamorous culture rests upon your
shoulders! The Parisian woman is compulsive about being
a winner. Second-best is never good enough. This attitude
can result in a lack of flexibility. Sometimes it would be
nice if she could lighten up a little. Perhaps she could take
a leaf from her Italian sister's book and develop *solarità*,
a sunnier, cheerful outlook and attitude.

Hurried

We *Parisiennes* always seem to be in hurry. But even when
we're in a rush, we won't be seen flustered.
We retain a *je ne sais quoi* of Parisian calm. "Everything
is under control, dahling!" We are in constant movement,
we're chic whirlwinds, we're dynamos, but at the same
time we're cool as cucumbers. Our day is packed with
work appointments, PTA meetings, and quick runs
to the supermarket, as well as high-society evenings.
Not to mention shopping tours, aquagym lessons,
the dentist, and yoga lessons.
Perched on five-inch heels, we scurry kitty-corner across
busy Paris streets instead of crossing at crosswalks.
We're sure of ourselves, so we park our subcompacts
wherever we feel like it. The main thing is to wind up

LINKS
• Attitude
• High Standards
• Melancholy
• Snob

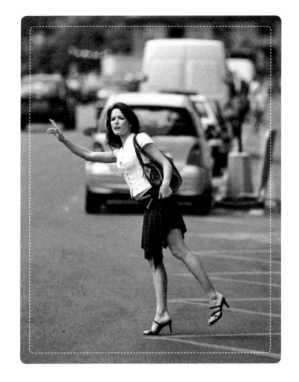

in the right place at the right time and not look ruffled! A Parisian's well-organized non-stop busy day! We're a little tired and stressed, but by the end we have done it all. Be careful that our "hyper-activity" is not, in reality, concealing "hyperactivity"—I mean, physical and mental.

Hyperactivity is a neurobiological disorder that affects a growing number of people (estimated at 5% of the population, adults and children), especially in large cities. In some countries, such as the United States and English-speaking Canada, hyperactivity is widespread, especially among entrepreneurs, politicians, and celebrities. In Europe, particularly in France, it is under-diagnosed and only recently recognized by the medical community. It is surely a question of tradition, beliefs, and culture.

Interiors

I have so often heard my foreign friends say, when entering my apartment, "It's so Parisian!" that I wanted to learn a bit more. Having recently visited dozens of Parisian apartments—from the living room to the bedrooms, from the dining room to the kitchen—and being reminded of the hundreds of others I have known throughout my life, I was able to find the common feature of all these Parisian interiors: a harmonious and skillfully proportioned blend of classic and contemporary. Like the Louvre and its pyramid, a good interior is a successful cohabitation of tradition and avant-garde creativity. It is due to the predisposition toward paradoxical combinations that Paris, one of the most romantic and classic cities in the world, has become the bulwark of contemporary art.

"Those who love the 6th arrondissement or the 7th arrondissement of Paris, aren't looking for Haussmann

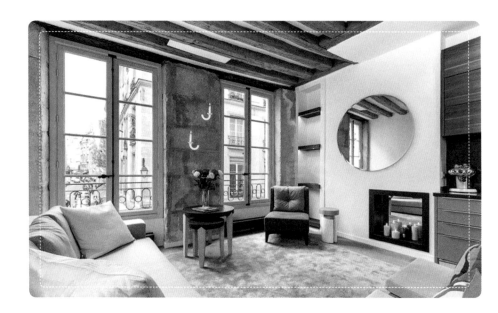

MY TIP
If you're lucky enough to have high ceilings, a fireplace, old parquet floors, and large English windows, just add designer furniture or beautiful objects and you're done. At least in part! Otherwise, before thinking about furniture, try to re-create this "Parisian" base with classic details such as ceiling moldings, wood paneling, glossy parquet flooring, a large antique mirror, long classic curtains in a single color, and so forth.

elegance but for seventeenth-century and eighteenth-century charm: old parquet floors, fireplaces, and timbered ceilings. On the other hand, a lot of foreigners, especially North Americans, purchase places needing renovation and do a contemporary makeover, sometimes even covering up the antique wooden beams."
Thierry Chomel de Varagnes, Associated Director of Barnes International

On the other hand, Parisian furnishings strongly transmit the personality of their owners, especially their history. The furniture of families with a wealth of memories and curious objects is mixed with photographs and beautiful modern objects. Woe to the interior designer who tells a Parisian woman that her grandmother's Boulle table has no place in their design! "Madame" is sentimental and has an innate sense of aesthetics, which can be seen in the furnishings of her home. She puts her soul into creating interiors capable of arousing emotions. Every object has its place and contributes to the overall balance. In this frantic search for perfection, the lighting is fundamental (apartments are often dark, except those on the top floor)—a skillful mix of natural light filtered by curtains and veils, table lamps, chandeliers, ceiling lamps, wall lamps, and, of course, candles! Attention: everything should be refined but functional. Every object must be useful, beautiful, and convey a certain dose of fantasy or emotion, otherwise it's out! Spare the gadgets, unless they were purchased at an antiques market or an art gallery. To sum up, though every Parisian interior is unique, each one conveys the impression of the French decorative-arts tradition tastefully reinvented to coexist with the design and art of our time.

Paris is full of lovely furniture shops, art galleries, antique dealers, flea markets, and large DIY department stores where you can buy everything you need. You can really enjoy furnishing a home; just follow these few basic rules and you're done.

- Mix old and new and also various styles. Never too much of anything; for interior design, less is more, as long as it's chic.
- Look for and buy vintage—that is what antiques and flea markets are for! No vulgarities or gadgets; only beautiful (and this does not necessarily mean expensive) and unique pieces and objects that have "soul."
- Leave the walls white, so that they can best perform their jewel-box function and optimize the light.
- Carefully plan the lighting of the dining room. It should gently enhance both your guests' faces and the food. No overly aggressive lighting.
- Pay attention to the smallest details of your table decorations, according to the same concept of mixing classic and modern.
- Think of flowers, white to be typically Parisian, or a single type—a large bouquet of peonies or tulips on the coffee table or even wildflowers, the kind "we just brought back from our Normandy country house."
- Don't overlook the smell of the apartment or of the house. Whether it comes from a freshly baked croissant, a fire in the fireplace, or a candle, it must be authentic and enjoyable, a kind of olfactory signature.

J

Jeans

The Parisian woman likes to consider HER pair of jeans (or pairs, and woe be it to anyone who touches them) a primary part of her wardrobe, so they are unsuitable for gardening, unless it's high-society gardening or the *jardins* of the Palace of Versailles. She wears them "casual chic" or "elegant cool," from morning to night, during the week or on the weekend, from the kitchen to the meeting room, at an opening in Saint-Germain-des-Prés or riding a bicycle through the streets of the French capital. Regardless of the cut or the color of her jeans, the Parisian woman will manage to find a way to show off her

MY TIP
You will never
see a Parisian woman
in low-rise jeans that
reveal a narrow thong
or a piercing and never
in a pair of jeans with
designs, embroidery,
or tears.

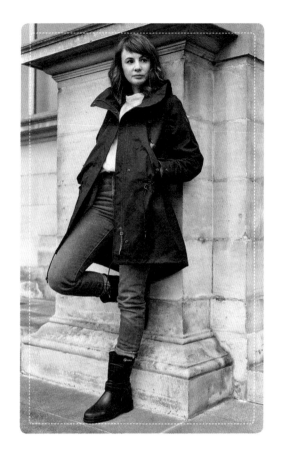

creativity and make them the centerpiece of her look. In Paris, jeans are mainly blue, black, white, or gray. If she is a fashion addict, she follows the latest trends to the letter, and the "certified" Parisian woman wears cigarette jeans: more elegant, that fit like a glove, and are therefore more feminine, but above all are more easily matched to tops and shoes of any style. This year, I love *Givenchy* and *A.P.C.* jeans. And my *Aigle's* (photo).

• For an even sexier, more feminine spirit, the Parisian woman will also wear slim-fits (if her shape allows it), because they make her look taller and give her a rock-chic touch (*Les Petites, Maje, Kookai*, or *Yves Saint-Laurent*). Pay attention to the volume rule of the chic silhouette:

slim-fit bottom = loose-fitting top (and vice versa).
• The wardrobe of a self-respecting Parisian woman must contain the trio of black, white, and navy jeans, plus a pair of light blue or faded jeans but ONLY if she looks good in them (in Paris the concept of aesthetics is fundamental and a Parisian woman wears only what looks good and enhances her: if light-colored jeans make her look fat, they're gone in a flash).
• Always with one eye on the classics and the other on the "must haves" (according to the press) of the season, the Parisian woman renewed her wardrobe this year with one or two pairs of trendy jeans: one flared for a gypsy-chic 1970s look (*Gérard Darel, Claudie Pierlot,* or *Leon & Harper*); one short or with the edges turned up, baring her ankles in a pair of ballerinas, Derbies, or high heels. And of course, she has a pair of "boyfriend" jeans that she wears with white *Stan Smith* or *Converse* sneakers. So Parisian!
• Very cute: navy jeans worn with heels and a tuxedo jacket with a stylish, sexy, and slightly see-through black top or with a lovely white blouse! It is one of my favorite evening outfits when traveling and when I'm sick of trying to accessorize my little black dress.
• As for white jeans, the Parisian woman wears them all year round, with a cream or gray cashmere sweater, a small silk top, a large red sweater, brown boots, a man's jacket, and so on. I love to wear them on the weekend with a navy sailor sweater and flat black moccasins. But they must have an impeccable cut (my favorite basic white jeans are signed *Loro Piana*) to avoid the "little Michelin man" effect of light jeans.
• But the stars of Paris are undoubtedly black jeans that she wears in ALL STYLES, with elegant *Roger Vivier* ballerinas, sandals, or high heels, or with boots and a leather jacket, or with a denim blouse. In short, they are one of the basic items always present in her wardrobe. My favorites: *The Kooples, Agnès B*, and *Comptoir des Cotonniers.*

Jewelry

While in other cultures "over accessorizing" is seen simply as a demonstration of femininity, in Paris it's considered good form not to overdo it for fear of looking tasteless. That might seem a paradoxical attitude, but it's based on the Parisian woman's mentality of "less is more." Basically, you can spoil a look by trying to overdo it, and that applies to jewelry, makeup, accessories, and plastic surgery. So:

• With something dressy, she'll wear super understated jewelry; bling isn't her thing. A little chain around her neck with a discreet pendant like a medal, a little cross, or a tiny diamond; a big one would be tasteless! On her fingers, a simple pretty ring or wedding band—not much fun but chic! She might add an equally simple bracelet like a gold

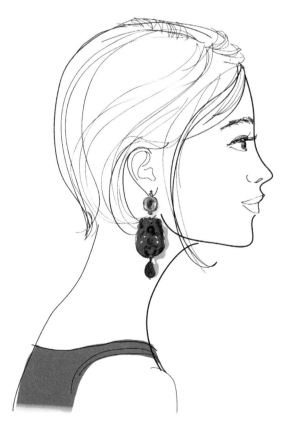

bangle, a lucky-charm bracelet on a cord given to her by her children or brought back from holiday, or an elegant chain to go with her classic young girl's watch (her jewelry often consists of items symbolizing an event in her life: her eighteenth birthday, her wedding, her First Communion) or a chunky man's watch. She also loves necklaces with pearls and semiprecious stones and antique earrings inherited from her grandmother or bought at an antique shop. If her evening dress is plain, then she might wear jewelry that is flashier but still elegant. Jewelry by Italian designers such as *Michela Bruni Reichlin* (illustration) or contemporary artists such as *Shourouk* is really in now.

• During the day the Parisian woman can adopt a simple look without artifice or jewelry, never denying her femininity. And the next day she can abandon her almost pathological simplicity and wear bigger or more prominent jewelry, provided that her dress is casual. She'd be too afraid of looking blingy! Contrasting styles is her favorite game: she'll wear super sophisticated or designer earrings with a cashmere turtleneck, and a diamond necklace with a slim-fit denim shirt or a white T-shirt. The Parisian woman doesn't like junk, so we're talking about quality jewelry here (remember, quality doesn't necessarily mean expensive) or exclusive or fashionable finds (she loves the idea of "exclusive pieces"), whether they're worth a lot or not, but never imitations; she's allergic to "counterfeit." Her culture and education have taught her to love the "genuine article," its intrinsic value and the creativity behind it. Given her borderline snobby personality, wearing a counterfeit is a terrible *faux pas* in Paris; better to wear something that's genuine and unknown than something that's known but a forgery!

• What to wear with your LBD? "For me, beautiful pearls are always super elegant and never dated, representing timeless Parisian chic. A pearl necklace and earrings with your little black dress looks great, classic but so chic."
Joëlle, Place de la Concorde, February 10

L

Language

Not only does the Parisian woman have the gift of gab, she also has her own language. I mean a repertoire of trendy expressions that may contain refined language, Franglais, or even slang picked up from her teenage prodigy. Her speech must be classy yet fashionable, with just the right touch of Parisian snootiness. Colorful language, indeed, but not always easy to follow. And if you miss even one word, you might miss the best part of her story. Your new Parisian friend may not show her impatience to your face, but behind your back ... goodness me!

The true *Parisienne* is witty and ironic but never vulgar. If she has been well schooled and properly brought up, she will put people at ease with witty, tactful, and charming speech. In fact, for many a Parisian, language is the starting point of seduction. If she is interested in a guy (and vice versa), he'll never forget his first conversation with her. What she says and how she says it are carefully crafted to beguile. The Parisian woman speaks her mind. Whereas in Anglo-American cultures, "politically correct" is a must, the French woman just says what she thinks. Not only are you allowed to speak your mind here, it's actually expected of you (as long as you're courteous,

juste incroyable

j'adore ∞ TROP MOCHE

Un truc de fou!

MY TIP
How to talk like a *Parisienne?* First of all, sound like you know what you're talking about. There has to be some substance to what you say. Talk about the headlines or culture. Make your point with anecdotes and a touch of humor. No shaggy-dog stories. Be captivating. Don't be a drag. And try using some of the cool expressions shown here (remember to D-R-A-G out the syllables in caps).

of course). Genteelly hurting people's feelings is part of Frenchness. Moreover, the French, you know, are not only people of character, with a temperament that focuses on appearances and theatrical effect; the French are also, and above all, interested in expressing themselves and, obviously, having freedom of speech.

- *C'est ZSHOOOste incroyABLE* (Incredible!). She's telling the scoop of the century and you're dying to hear what comes next.
- *C'est un TRUC de fou.* (It was insane, nuts, screwed up, ridiculous!) For example, how long she had to wait in line at *Ladurée.*
- *C'est une signature.* To talk about a distinctive piece of designer jewelry or a unique dish by a famous chef; a masterpiece that anyone who knows anything can recognize a mile away.
- *Je trouve ça EXTRAordinaire.* Whenever you want to show interest in whatever you are talking about.
- *Ça c'est MAAgnifique* (It's magnificent!). Same sort of thing as above but more definitive. What else can you say?
- *C'est une pièce YOUUU-nique.* If you're Parisian, you're mad about limited editions and singular objects. Something to say about a sculpture at a *vernissage* or a *Chanel* bag.
- *Tu m'étonnes!* Sounds like "you astonish me" but really means just the opposite. "You are SO right! I couldn't agree more!"
- *Ça, J'AAH-dore.* Used to describe a cult object or the latest skincare treatment at a trendy spa.
- *Ça c'est SUUUperbe.* May be uttered several times at a chic boutique, but best used when the shop assistant shows you just the little dress you've been looking for— then you can give the expression appropriate oomph!
- *C'est juste AAAllucinant quoi.* In-fucking-credible!
- *C'est TROOHHHp moche!* (Grosses me out!) Used to decry a failed facelift or a miniskirt on someone who was deemed too old to be wearing it.

La Ville Lumière

Have you ever wondered why Paris is called *La Ville Lumière* (City of Light)? Dine early and go for a walk to discover the city's nighttime face—a dazzling, almost surreal vision; a beautiful girl who at night turns into a charming woman bedecked with precious jewels. The metaphor is not perfect, but at dusk the city is transformed into a grand spectacle of light, absolutely not to be missed. We Parisians are accustomed to it, but we are always thrilled by the genius of the engineers, "magicians" who study architectural works down to the smallest details in order to enhance them with LEDs and beams of light. Have you seen the capital's monuments exalted by blazing lights? Follow a trail of lights from the Grand Palais to the Pyramide du Louvre, from the Musée des Beaux-Arts to the cathedral of Notre-Dame to discover the lighting that promotes the beauty of Paris's cultural heritage. I love the windows of the Musée d'Orsay illuminated to enhance its early twentieth-century building and the Assemblée Nationale, clothed in its blue dress, a symbol of peace. Observe, with all the necessary calm, the skillful lighting of Paris's bridges, a play of shadows on the stone and sculptures, specifically created to enhance their majesty

LINKS
• Marianne
• Rive Gauche, Rive Droite
• Tour Eiffel

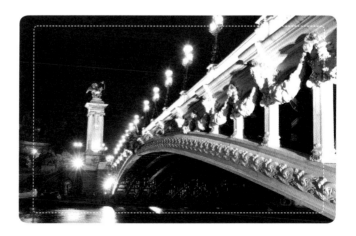

and uniqueness. Lighting that exalts the details. Less famous than the glitter of the Tour Eiffel, the illuminated Parisian signs are nevertheless sublime, whether steady or flashing, with their multicolored neon letters against the dark sky. But it is during the year-end holidays that the *Ville Lumière* gives its best, with its avenues and squares dressed in wonderful lights, the spectacular windows of its department stores, and Christmas trees set up everywhere (you should absolutely see the one in *Galeries Lafayette* with its 5,000 lit ornaments).

Lingerie

If we've said it once, we've said it a dozen times: the Parisian woman is a paradox. She says she prefers classic lingerie, all satin and lace, but she also dares to try sexy underthings, just for fun, to titillate the fancy. In fact, she has a very liberated way of dressing, within the limits of Parisian elegance and harmony of style. Who better than she can wear borderline "naughty" things yet remain stylish and classy? The *Parisienne* loves good-girl lingerie but she can also dress up like a temptress and somehow preserve a well-bred, good-girl look. Her secrets? Let me tell you two:
• She softens a hard style with more classic items. For example, if she wears a black lace bra (that she certainly didn't inherit from her grandmother), she'll wear a plain white blouse over it for a tactful yet troubling see-through effect. The result is provocative but refined.
• She has the restraint to wear no more than one sexy thing at a time. If she's in the mood to wear a panther print bustier (Lord, have mercy!), she'll refrain from wearing scarlet lipstick and a miniskirt. She'll wear nude makeup, plain blue jeans, and a tailored black jacket. These things are ultra-classic but will look sexy with the bustier. Elegant black heels will be the finishing touch to a look that says, "Provocative but well behaved."

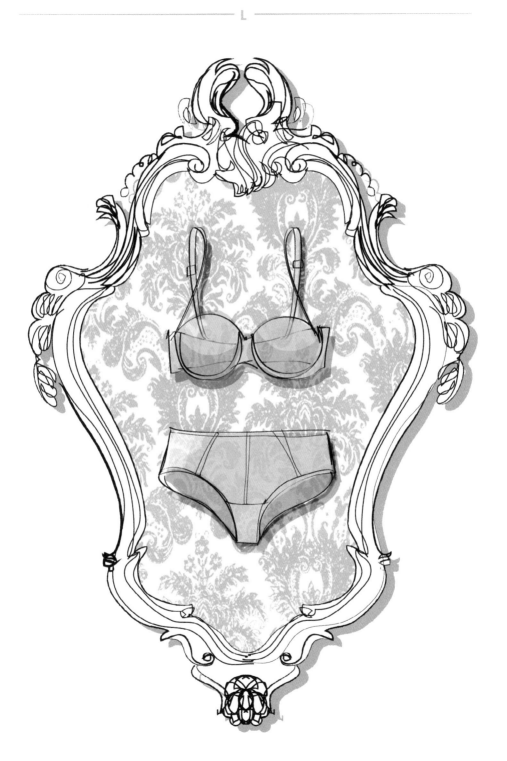

In sum, if you've got it, flaunt it, but only with class and charm. You can't be crude or lurid. Whether you prefer demure *Petit Bateau* panties or *Dita Von Teese*'s vintage undies, French lingerie is always charming.

The relationship between the sexy Parisian woman and lingerie has evolved over time. Today women who show off their sexy underwear no longer risk being seen as an object of desire. More than to seduce, the Parisian woman buys underwear for herself, to make her feel like a woman but also for her own pleasure. By the way, she also likes to offer her best friends lingerie as a gift.

Little Black Dress

MY TIP
Study your shape and be merciless—a little black dress worn badly is a mistake, not too short or too long, not tight or low-cut, if it doesn't flatter you. There is nothing more depressing, so be reasonable and find the LBD that works for you. And that means trying them on and being objective. Having ten black dresses, even from the big names, that don't fit you is the same as not having any! As a general rule: no super frou-frou princess dresses—not in Paris.

We've said, and it's true, that we Parisian women love "little" black dresses, which we call *petites robes noires*. In Paris, the adjective *petite* has the connotation "affectionate and refined." My American friends are always telling me, "Going to dinner in Paris means seeing 99% of the women dressed in all types of black dresses." Even if we collect them, there's always one missing—it's almost pathological. Skin-tight, long-sleeved, low-cut, in vaporous silk, short, elegant, rock ... in short, having five to ten is the minimum for the Parisian woman's wardrobe.

How to choose one? Just think about different situations and above all don't always buy the same model. It doesn't make sense to buy five short-sleeved + backless + knee-length styles, if you don't have at least one long-sleeved + elegant + high-necked for an evening at the Opéra Bastille and a long one to wear with low sandals at an elegant cocktail party on the Rive Gauche. The Parisian is rational, so why complicate your life with a magnificent and expensive turquoise dress that, from its first wearing will be known and recognized by everyone and will go out of fashion in a month, while, with the same style in black, you can accessorize it differently fifty times and no one will ever realize it. It's simple: in Paris or elsewhere, the black

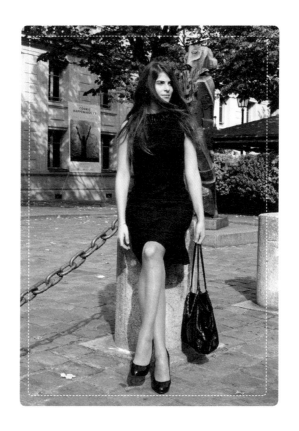

dress is elegant. Sexxxxxy. It makes all women beautiful!
A *must have* that lends itself to endless combinations. Of
course, there's always our grandmother to tell us we're
too young to dress in mourning, or that black makes us
look "pale," and our boyfriend who thinks a black dress is
very sexy on other women but he's "a bit tired of seeing
it on you," but apart from that, for us the little black dress
has no faults, only advantages. Coco Chanel helped us
a lot when in 1920 she created what Americans call the
LBD. Today, every fashion house and the most prestigious
brands have at least one or two styles of black dress,
something that opens up a very interesting hunting
season on Saturdays! Let's go find the perfect LBD!
By the way, this year, the *robe portefeuille* (or "wrap dress")

will be all the rage. First fashionable in the 1970s, it made a big comeback last summer. I found a really nice one on *La Redoute* website.

Where and how to wear the Little Black Dress in Paris?
• Dinner downtown (simplicity and elegance, especially if you do not know the context).
• Opening (dare with an extra touch of sexy—but not too much—ballerina shoes, and a big bag).
• Stylish restaurant (attention to accessories—remember that only your bust will be seen, so it's useless to buy a dress whose main feature is the cut of the back).
• Elegant cocktail party (be tall and sophisticated! Heels and a skin-tight dress).
• Family reunion (go classic with a pastel cardigan to please grandma).
• Theater (think about post-theater plans, so wear a cardigan that you can take off—two dresses in one).
• Evening tête-à-tête with the boyfriend (don't overdo it, no plunging necklines on the first date).
• Exclusive Paris club (*Interallié, Tir aux Pigeons, Automobile Club de France, Country Club, Polo*, etc.). In general go very chic and classic (no plunging necklines and not skin-tight).
Pay attention to your hairstyle: a classic bun can be very elegant on a model but it could make you look old. If in doubt, ask your daughter or your cousin's daughter if it works for you. In summer, during the day, wear your LBD with oversize sunglasses, a man's jacket, and a large tote bag, and you'll be perfect for circulating in the capital's outdoor cafés. My current favorites: *Yves Saint-Laurent, Givenchy, Balenciaga, Carven, Roland Mouret,* and *Nina Ricci.* More affordable: *Vanessa Bruno, A.P.C., Isabel Marant, Gérard Darel,* and *Zadig & Voltaire.* In Paris, there are very interesting models from *Monoprix* and in many more inexpensive downtown boutiques. Just choose the right accessories and check the quality of the fabric and finish. All are appropriate for life in Paris—*chic* and *shock!*

Luxury

Luxury products have a soul—ours, but especially that of their creators. For the Parisian woman, they are synonymous with beauty, emotion, and creativity and satisfy the need to escape and dream—so necessary for her equilibrium, like the air she breathes. It's not the brand or the price that interests her but the poetry of the object, whether an engagement ring from *Van Cleef & Arpels,* an evening dress from *Christian Dior Couture,* or a tuxedo jacket from *Yves Saint-Laurent*, dishes from *Bernardaud,* silverware from *Christofle,* a vase from *Lalique* or *Daum,* a bottle of vintage *Krug* champagne, *Baccarat* crystal

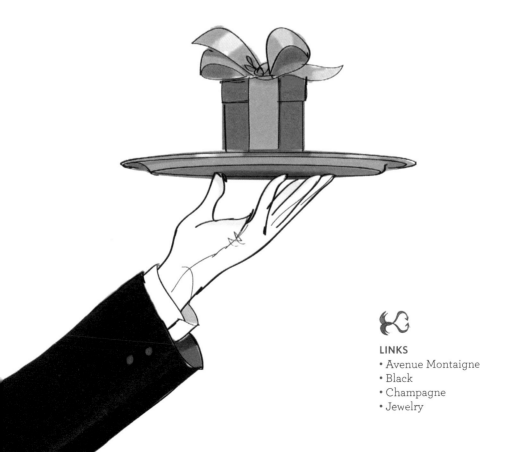

LINKS
• Avenue Montaigne
• Black
• Champagne
• Jewelry

glasses, embroidered sheets from *D. Porthault,* a *Hermès* wallet, or even a dish by chef *Alain Ducasse.* Even if they are sometimes unaffordable, all these beautiful objects are part of the dream imagery that the Parisian woman will try to make reality when the occasion allows. They are a kind of investment in beauty and quality, that will embellish her daily life or special moments of her life, because the Parisian woman loves to be surrounded by beautiful objects that give satisfaction and emotion. Wearing well-tailored clothing thrills and reassures her; having nice dishes or bed and table linens from a great designer is a real treat for her.

Each luxury item is considered a work of art that contributes to her zest for life. But for her, real luxury is the designers who have a history that she is as proud of as if it were her own. *Christofle* or *Baccarat* are always present on the table at her grandparents' lunches, and, for this reason, she will put *Christofle* or *Baccarat* on her wedding list because they are a value that provides confidence and never loses its class. Master glassmakers and engravers of proverbial skill, cabinet makers from the hand-crafted tradition, dressmakers, shoemakers—these and many others represent superior craftsmanship rich in culture and history that the Parisian respects as almost sacred. All these beautiful luxury brands remind us of our traditions: of fabricating objects of a quality that the entire world admires and that our children will always admire; of representing France's image in the world; of seducing by offering us genuine products of typically French good taste; and finally, and most importantly, of respect for a job well done. The true nobility of luxury is the beauty of the craftsman's gesture capable of achieving a quality and finish of unique execution. In this century, a period of excessive vulgarization and automation, one of the greatest merits of the creators of luxury is to maintain, against all odds, the highest level of craftsmanship. And that is what the Parisian woman loves. Long live true French luxury!

Macaroons

This fun, colorful, tasty little round cake makes Parisians crazy. They come in such a variety that the choice is a really hard task. There are macaroons with a thin crunchy outside, others with a praline shell. There are round macaroons and hamburger-shaped ones. They come in warm colors and flashy ones. Some macaroons have creamy centers and others soft hearts. Each Parisian pastry chef has his or her own recipe. Walking around Paris, it is impossible not to see them—they are everywhere!

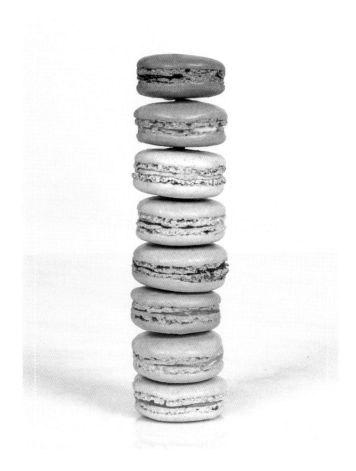

But which is the best? How can you choose? Do you really have to try'em all before you find the one you like the best? The macaroon is a subject that *Parisiennes* can never agree on: there are Parisians who will buy them only on the Rive Gauche and others who swear only by the Rive Droite. There are purists who prefer the not-too-sweet "to sublime natural flavors" at *Dalloyau*. There are unconditional fans of *Lenôtre,* where the macaroons are both soft and crunchy. The fashionistas go to *Pierre Hermé* to taste macaroons with innovative flavors such as *crème brulée*—vanilla with caramel chips. Connoisseurs flock to *Arnaud Larher* to experience the different textures. There are those faithful to *Gérard Mulot,* the macaroon chef of the stars, who bakes a soft and crunchy macaroon with a delicate taste. Then there are moms who bake their own macaroons with the kids after school.

Macaroons have become an incredible hit. They are conceived practically like the finest French wines. Nary a tourist leaves Paris without a snapshot of the Tour Eiffel ... and a box of macaroons. The best traditional macaroons are said to come from *Ladurée* (photo). My favorite? *Fleur de sel* caramel, a classic and a *Ladurée* specialty. Ever been to their new store on Rue de Castiglione? You must! It's the *ne plus ultra* in gourmet macaroons.

Madeleine

What do you think is a typical name for a *Parisienne?* Well, I suppose it depends on when you were born. Lola, Sarah, and Alice are still playing in the sandbox. Noémie, Jade, and Léa are high school seniors and will need to mature a little before they consolidate their Parisian style. As for us, their elders Béatrice, Caroline, Isabelle, Marion, and Sophie, we're all proud specimens of today's Parisian woman. And then there's Madeleine ... Madeleine is our grandmother, a super Parisian, modern, lively, and elegant in her pencil skirt, her pearls, and her navy top. We all

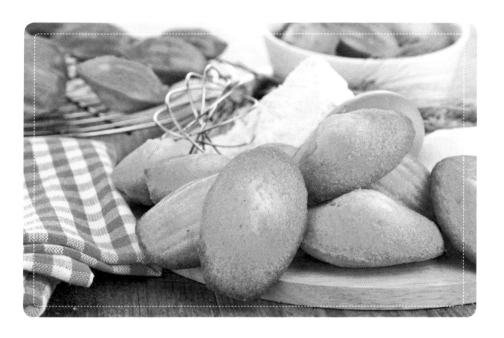

MY TIP
Notice the wonderful
fragrance coming from
your oven, a smell like
no other. Concentrate
hard on a special feeling
or a pleasant image. Try
and associate the
madeleine smell with
those special thoughts,
and see if those
thoughts come back to
you the next time you
enjoy this Parisian treat.

have a Granny Madeleine, one of the most popular girl's
names from 1930 until about 1950. Granny Madeleine
is our muse. She hasn't always gotten along well with her
daughter, who was something of a revolutionary in her
day, but we, her granddaughters, take inspiration from
her style, values, and *art de vivre*. Her enthusiasm and
imagination are literally in our DNA.

For we Parisians, the name Madeleine also evokes writer
Madeleine de Scudéry (1607–1701), the guru of French
seduction who invented an imaginary country called
"Tender," a land of courtly and platonic love, where
amorous discourse turned into games of wits. Madeleine
also denotes a famous square in the heart of Paris
with its marvelous church that looks so lovely lit up
at night. It's funny how the Madeleine church is said to
be "typically Parisian," when in reality, with its massive
columns, its architecture is reminiscent of ancient Greece.
Paradoxical as a *Parisienne*! And then we cannot say
the name Madeleine without thinking of our beloved

Granny's Madeleines

For a batch of 16 madeleines
2 eggs
1/3 cup sugar
3/4 cup flour
1 tbsp. orange blossom water
1 pinch yeast
3 1/2 tbsp. melted butter
1 3/4 tbsp. milk

THE RECIPE
The secret to making a good madeleine is the mold: it has to be high in quality, made of silicone or metal. What's the difference? If you use a silicone mold the madeleine will be lighter in color. I prefer to use a metal mold (always butter it): the unmistakable "bump" of the madeleine will come out perfectly.

Melt the butter over low heat in a saucepan and set aside. Mix the eggs with the sugar to form a consistent mix (it should be intense white in color, otherwise the madeleines won't rise when baked and will be heavy). Add the orange blossom water, a little milk, the yeast, and the butter. Add more milk as necessary to obtain a smooth batter. Let the batter set for 15 minutes. Preheat the oven to 450°F. Butter the madeleine molds and fill them carefully with batter, since the madeleines are going to rise. Bake for about 5 minutes and then lower the temperature to 400°F. Bake another 10 minutes or until the madeleines are golden brown. Remove the madeleines from their molds as soon as you take them out of the oven.

author Marcel Proust. His madeleine is not a woman but a famous mini cake of the same name. When the narrator dips his madeleine into a cup of tea, the taste brings back childhood memories. This metaphor is often used in France to evoke anything that awakens long-forgotten feelings.

And so, last but not least, a madeleine is a sweet little French cake with a unique taste that's very popular in French tearooms. It's a French specialty we all learn to bake at a tender age.

Makeup

I'd like to bring up a taboo subject: the Parisian would like the whole wide world to find her naturally gorgeous, which would imply that she never wore any make up at all! "Her cheeks? Naturally pink because she has the complexion of a country lass." But of course! "Her lips are oh-so-red from eating organic berries and sipping fine French wine." Yeah, sure!

Not so long ago, one of my girlfriends, Ann from Walnut Creek, was saying to me, "You use so little makeup." I got a kick out of that because I spend at least half an hour every morning putting on my war paint, and once I've finished I have to check myself out in every mirror in the house to see if my makeup is invisible in every kind of light. Actually, I don't want people to notice my makeup. I just want to give my face a little mystical *je ne sais quoi*, hide a few of life's little imperfections, and show off my best features. I've done a quick survey of my friends and they all do the same thing. Could makeup be the best-kept secret in Paris? *Mais bien sur*! Makeup? *Moi*? I look this way naturally, even straight out of bed!

Personally, I've picked up a few tips from the pros (dermatologists, makeup artists, nutritionists), and I try to put their advice into practice every day.

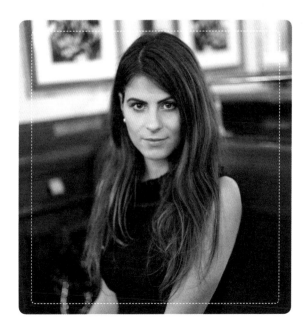

LINKS
- Nails
- Plastic Surgery
- Seduction

- My makeup session starts by drinking a big glass of water to hydrate my skin from the inside. Then I apply moisturizing cream with a smoothing effect.
- Next comes the camouflage job. Spots, dark circles, and aging shadows have to be "corrected." My skincare product for this has to be the right consistency (not too wet and not too dry) and match my skin color 100% (never darker). Next, I fill in little wrinkles around my mouth and eyes. I apply a little *Kiehl's*, which I find more subtle than *MAC*.
- Then the "real" makeup can start. I must sculpt and enhance! For the evening, I put on a very light foundation, like a light-diffusing *Guerlain* in a natural beige color. Then I add a touch of *Estée Lauder*'s light *Night Repair Eye* gel to the eye contour, near my nose. For the daytime, no foundation, but a light powder like *Diorlight*, which I've been using since the age of sixteen!
- On my lids, a natural eye shadow, never pearly, as a base for a pair of natural beiges to bring out my eyes. For an evening out, I might go for something a little darker but always subtly elegant. On my lashes, I wear quality mascara but never too much and only on the top lashes. I use a comb to separate them and then an eyelash curler. In the summer, like many of my friends, I use a little eyelash dye to settle the mascara problem for swimming.
- For a youthful look, I use *Bourgeois Rose Coup de Foudre* (I've always loved their fragrance).
- For my lips, I first put on a good coat of *Nivea* lip balm. Then, for daytime, I apply a simple, glossy peach, strawberry, or transparent *Clinique* or *L'Oréal* lipstick. At night, I wear a more provocative red if I'm in a flirty mood. Since the *Parisienne* is never supposed to overdo anything, when I wear red lipstick I attenuate it with a Kleenex. I might wear red lipstick during the day but only for a casual chic look with jeans and a cardigan! These days I'm never without my *Opéra* lipstick by Dior. It's sublime and feels so nice.

• The eyebrows are slightly plucked, and, once again, exaggeration is not elegant. I brush on a dark beige eye shadow just a shade darker than my natural skin color. *Voilà!* There you go. And if, despite all this artistry, a few tiny wrinkles remain, it's no big deal, right? They're just little signs of my personality, and I'm proud of them and ready to face the world. Am I French or not?

Oh, I almost forgot. I always carry around a mini makeup pouch for a little rearview-mirror touchup work. But you'll never catch me touching up my makeup in public!

LINKS
• Children
• Language
• Madeleine
• Vintage

Marianne

It's impossible not to mention Marianne, one of the most famous French women. The allegorical figure of the Republic, the icon of democracy! The woman who embodies the French values contained in *Liberté, Egalité,*

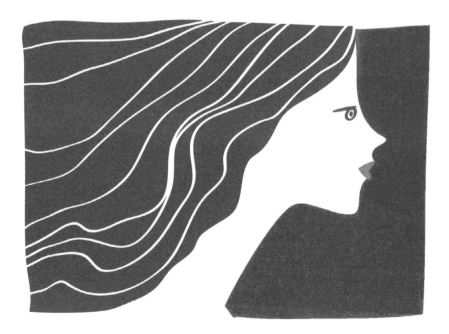

Fraternité. Today not always respected, as she should be, you will find her anywhere—on stamps, coins, in town halls, government buildings, and French embassies scattered in every corner of the world. Did you know that it was Marianne de Lamartine, muse and wife of the poet Alphonse de Lamartine, who, for the first time, in the early nineteenth century, gave her bust to the Republic?

Today, though there is no official model for Marianne, the most popular representations are those that use the faces of famous women. In the 1970s Brigitte Bardot and Michele Morgan lent their faces to Marianne, then it was the turn of Catherine Deneuve and Inès de la Fressange in 1989. Laetitia Casta played Marianne at the beginning of the twenty-first century and Sophie Marceau in 2012. Who do you think will be next?

Marinière

Ask a young Parisian to draw a woman, and chances are she'll sketch one wearing a *marinière!* A *marinière* is a blue-striped, long-sleeved jersey inspired by French Navy shirts. It is so ingrained in our culture that it could practically become our national uniform. Today, all the big name brands have their own *marinière*, and there seem to be an infinite number of versions. Nonetheless, the Parisian tends to prefer high-quality traditional dark blue and white models made in France by *Petit Bateau*, *Saint James*, or *Lux Armor.*

MY TIP
If you want to avoid Brittany beachwear and make your outfit more Parisian, try wearing your *marinière* under a black smoking jacket or a man's tailored jacket. Or wear it over black leather leggings or a pair of jeans. Add accessories to make it dressier and mix styles. Parisian seduction: wear a red or black lace bra under your *marinière* with a strap showing nonchalantly on one shoulder. In summer it looks fabulous with shorts and rhinestone sandals —on well-manicured feet, of course— for a true Parisian look!

HISTORY

When Coco Chanel was seen wearing a *marinière* between the two world wars, the blue striped top soon became an icon of French elegance and part of our cultural heritage. In 1960 Yves Saint-Laurent was the first to transform the simple *marinière* into a work of haute couture. Jean-Paul Gautier made the *marinière* fashionable again in the 1980s, and Sonia Rykiel glamorized it with her basic white and blue version in 2000. In 2011 Colette, the high priestess of Parisian fashion (unfortunately, her legendary boutique on Rue Saint-Honoré has now been closed), dedicated part of her boutique to *marinières* by *Chanel, Comme des Garçons, Hermès,* and other big-name designers. The *marinière* has since been consecrated as a "noble" garment and can now be seen on catwalks next to the legendary "little black dress." It is the classic top worn by the in-crowd. Just as no French meal is complete without French bread, the Parisian's wardrobe is incomplete without its *marinière*. This summer, the *marinière* was everywhere, in every collection, so get one now. I've found a *marinière* by *Leon & Harper* that's just too cute and one by *Chanel* that I absolutely adore. *Gérard Darel* and *Promod* have *marinières* that you'll love, too.

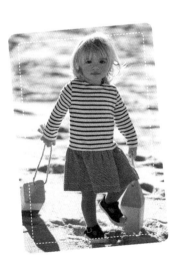

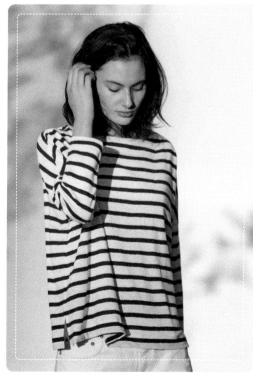

Market

The Parisian loves to buy healthy foods that are rich in vitamins to cook over the weekend. Fresh, healthy food is a good way to pamper yourself, get your weight under control, and soothe the tummy you so mistreated during the week, when you skipped meals or gulped down sandwiches while rushing off to business meetings and appointments with your beautician. She wants to be a socially responsible shopper. At *le marché* (not a grocery store but a good old-fashioned farmers' market), she buys local, seasonal products (except for goji berries and other health foods that we simply have to have all year round). The best time to visit the market is Sunday morning,

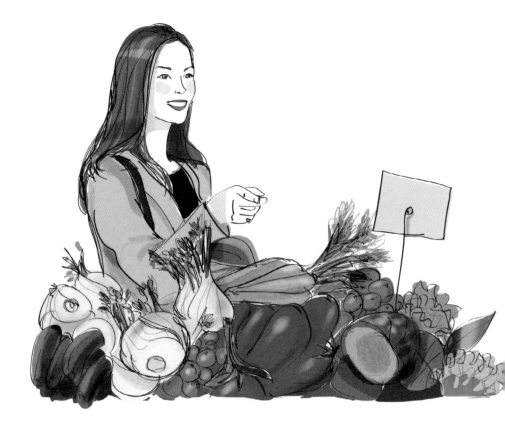

because that's when we have the most chance of running into girlfriends to share the latest gossip. I recommend *Raspail* marketplace on the Rive Gauche and the *President Wilson* marketplace in the vicinity of Place Trocadéro, Rive Droite. Some *Parisiennes* swear only by the *Grande Épicerie de Paris*, a prestigious fine foods market with only the best in fruit and vegetables.

Melancholy

Audrey and Brune are having a coffee at the *Bistrot de la Tour Eiffel*:
Audrey: "You ok?"
Brune: "Yeah . . ."
"You look kind of sad."
"No, I'm ok, really."
"A penny for your thoughts."
"I'm thinking about my grandmother who loved chocolates, about a call from Timothé, what Tudy told me about Clémence (unbelievable). I'm not thinking about anything special, my mind's just wandering, I guess."
"Didn't you say you were seeing Valentin at 3:00?"

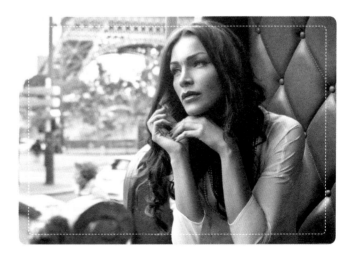

LINKS
• Attitude
• Grandma
• Grayness
• Hurried

"That's right. Why, what time is it now?"

"3:20."

"Oh my gosh! Gotta go. I'm wicked late. I'm so looking forward to seeing him."

Menu

The first time you see a Parisian woman looking at a menu in a restaurant, watch closely. She looks so damned focused that you'd swear she was cogitating on *War and Peace*! No, she's not concentrating on a graphic or literary analysis of said menu but pondering the quandary of balancing caloric intake against social grace. Dieting does you good, but refusing to partake in the joys of French cuisine is a social no-no. Here's a little insight if you want to act like a *Parisienne* at a restaurant.

• All Parisian girls are supposedly skinny. How do they do it? Do they live on just salad? Can't be, because a chic Parisian is expected to have a buttery croissant for breakfast, nibble fattening *saucisson* at cocktail time, and snack on gourmet macaroons. So what's the secret? In fact, each *Parisienne* does her own juggling act. My personal technique is "one yes for two no's." In other words, I spend one day enjoying the food I love, and then two days limiting myself to proteins, veggies, fruits, and nonfat dairy products. My friend Charlotte does two super "no's" then five "yes's" and my friend Chantal does one "yes" and then six "neither yes's nor no's." One thing's for sure: nothing would be sadder than 365 "yes's" or 365 "no's"!

• Parisian girls are said to be charming. Seated at the restaurant, she's deep in thought. "Is this a 'yes' day or a 'no' day?" Sooner or later the thought process comes to the question, "Who's sitting across from me?" which translates into, "Who do I have to charm? My grandmother, a guy I don't know that well, a girlfriend from the office, a bunch of buddies, my husband?"

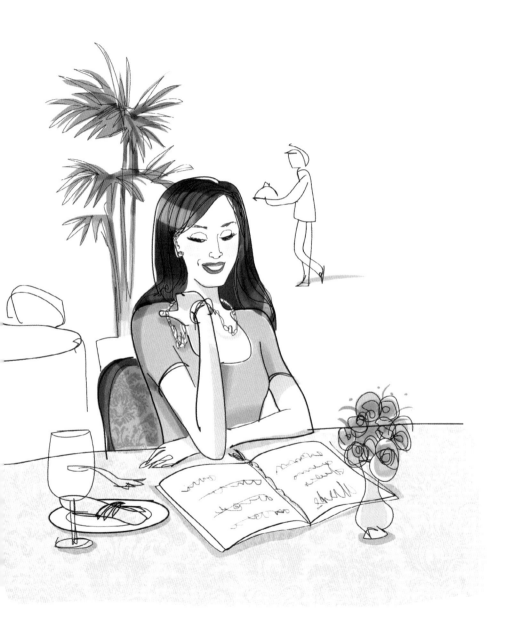

- If it's Grandma: I'm going to order a regional specialty from her part of France. It'll make her happy and she'll think I'm eating "right."
- If it's some guy: He's probably judging me. Pigging out is out of the question, but it would look just as bad not to enjoy having a meal with him. French men appreciate the company of a woman who likes a nice meal. No Frenchman is ever going ask you out twice if he hears, "No thanks, I'm on a diet" or if you order a plate of grilled vegetables if he takes you to a five-star restaurant.
- If it's a girlfriend from the office: either I chow down on something *gourmand* (ultra-fattening) just to make her jealous ("How can that bitch eat rich food like that and still fit into that dress?!") or I watch my weight like a good girl and just order salad.
- If it's my man: neither piggery nor starvation diet; a nice balanced dinner. Sometimes organic foods, sometimes we experiment. "The couple that eats together stays together."
- If I'm alone: it all depends on whether it's a "yes" day or a "no" day!

Museum

A true Parisian has a duty to know her city and its secrets. Always in a hurry, but curious and hungry for culture, she rarely misses the great exhibitions of the moment. *Musée d'Orsay, Palais de Tokyo, Quai Branly*, the *Louvre* ... she keeps an eye on the cultural agenda and follows it. At lunchtime, she waits in line to see the Joan Miró exhibition at the *Grand Palais*, wouldn't dream of missing the Egon Schiele show at the *Fondation Louis Vuitton*, and, on the weekend, takes her kids to discover the masterpieces of French heritage throughout Paris. If she doesn't have time, grandma will take the grandchildren to the museum because they have to begin appreciating art at a very young age! And if she needs to relax after a day of work, the Parisian woman

LINKS
- Parenting
- Rive Gauche, Rive Droite
- Roofs

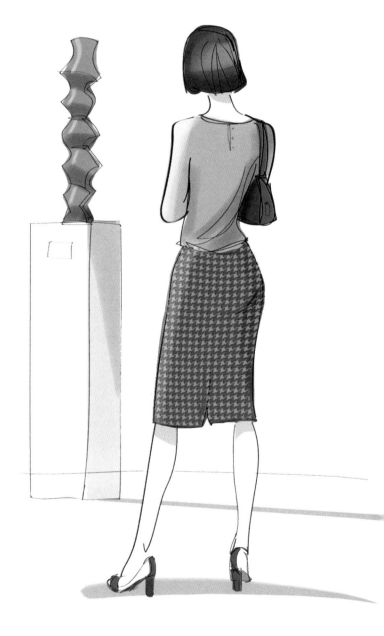

MY TIP
The *Nissim de Camondo, Carnavalet, Bourdelle,* and *Chasse et de la Nature* museums; the house of *Balzac*, the *Fondation Le Corbusier,* the *Cognacq-Jay Museum* ... Paris is full of wonderful museums that are little known but very interesting.

gladly grants herself a cultural evening in one of the many museums open at night (*Jacquemart-André* is open on Mondays until 8:30; the *Fondation Cartier* until 10:00 on Tuesdays, the fashion museum *Palais Galliera,* Thursdays until 9:00, etc.).

Mussels

Eating mussels like a *Parisienne* is an end in and of itself! Here's what my friends Charles from Boston and Carlo from Rome say:
"I'll try and explain it to you but the best thing would be to invite a Parisian woman out to dinner, as I did, in one of the capital's many seafood restaurants. Beware, influencing a Parisian woman is a tough job, but gently suggest that she orders the famous *moules marinières,*

LINKS
• Attitude
• Eating Right
• Wine

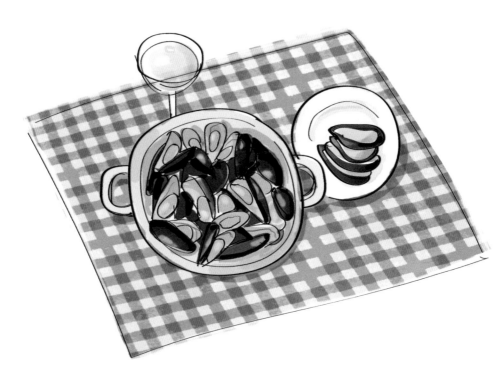

served in the traditional pot. Conversation will be easy and varied, because the Parisian woman knows how to conduct herself in company. The white wine will be dry, fresh, and pleasant and then the mussels arrive! Now watch and learn the method."
Charles, Boston, Hudson St., January 5

"The *Parisienne* has a very particular and feminine way of eating mussels. She selects a mussel and holds it delicately between her thumb and index finger. Thanks to the elasticity of the hinge, she's going to use it like a pincer. Then she takes another mussel with her left hand and uses the 'pincer' to remove the flesh of the mussel and bring it to her mouth. All with the nonchalance of a princess! She then puts the empty shell delicately on a plate that the waiter will have placed next to her, takes another mussel in her left hand, and repeats the process: extraction with the pincer shell, putting the mussel in her mouth ... What does she do with this second empty shell? No, she doesn't just dump it in the pot like 98% of the people all over the world. She slips the second shell into the first one and so on for all the mussels she eats! In the end, she'll have a real work of art on her plate—a harmonious composition of columns of empty shells, one inside the other. Such incredible sophistication! A spectacle to be seen and copied!"
Carlo, Rome, Via Veneto, January 15

N

Nails

The Parisian goes for a "good girl" look down to her nails. Even if she's moving to another house, her nails stay well manicured. Natural, nude, or red, the rule in Paris is "always chic, never cheap," even if the allure of the latest nail art fad and novel nail polishes is hard to resist. Cosmetics makers and fashion experts might want to convince you otherwise, but here's what some

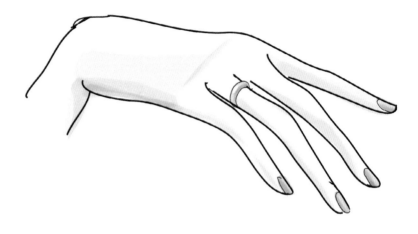

typical Parisians have to say about truly elegant hands.
• NO to inch-long claws: "They're inelegant and
aggressive. A real *Parisienne* would never wear them
like that. A few men might find them attractive, but not
we Parisians; they're too animal."
Cécile, Place de la Concorde, February 12
• YES to short, clean, natural nails. "A refined, well-
manicured lady is a winner in Paris. If you wear polish,
immaculate hands with natural or pinkish beige works
best in all circumstances."
Capucine, Avenue Mozart, March 20
• NO to sloppy nail polish. "There are women who will
slap on four or five coats of polish to avoid having to
completely redo their nails. That's the kind of detail that
kills style. And frankly, nail polish painted on hurriedly,
standing up in the metro, is yucky. When a Parisian is
short of time, she puts on transparent polish. You put on
color right or not at all."
Ambre, Place d'Auteuil, March 12
• NO to freaky nail art. "Nail care means fresh, delicate
hands, not theatrical paint. Nail art is cover girl stuff.
No way do I want to see it on the woman in my life!"
Antonin, Place de l'Opéra, January 13

• YES to a glossy topcoat. "I love it. It brightens up my hands, especially in the summer sun, on the beach with a tan!"
Clarisse, Rue François 1er, March 15
• NO to loud colors. "Flashy nails gross guys out, even if they're supposed to be the latest thing."
Romain, Avenue Gabriel, January 11
• YES to classic red. "Red nail polish, when it's well applied, is refined and sexy. Women like it and men like it! Looks great with everything, but I love it with a casual, 'jeans and trench coat' look. Even teens are crazy about it these days!"
Anaïs, TV reporter, December 15
• NO to the French manicure. "Funny isn't it? The one place where you don't do it is France! It isn't French, anyway. It's a technique that was developed for Hollywood actresses in the 1970s and called 'French' just to make it sound classier. Calling something 'French' is supposed to be automatically chic!"
Cindy, real estate broker, February 20
• YES to the natural manicure. "Polish and file your nails, remove cuticles and hydrate your hands and nails. The Parisian often keeps a second coat of polish for little touch-ups on the second and third day."
Jessica, beautician, Trocadéro, January 5

Oysters

My American girlfriend Pamela asked me to talk about French oysters. First of all, my view is this: though many countries produce oysters, not one in the world can offer a more complete "oyster-gastronomic" experience than France! Ordering oysters in Paris not only means eating oysters. It also means entering a world of *savoir vivre* and of *savoir faire*. Regardless of how the oysters are served, the French who are serving you want to make you feel privileged to be able to eat the most delicious oysters

LINKS
• Gastronomy
• Mussels
• The Best
• Wine

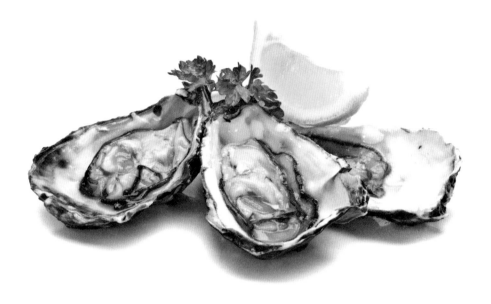

HISTORY
In Roman times, the French coast was where the first oysters were found. In modern times, France was the first country in Europe to start the cultivation of oysters on a large scale. It's called "oyster farming" and the oyster farmers are called *parqueurs*.

in the world. In France, especially Paris, oysters are not considered just any old shellfish. We serve some of the best oysters in the world, and they are considered a luxury food, worthy of respect. Dear Pamela, the *Ville Lumière* is a paradise for lovers of oysters! Oysters are flown in daily from Brittany or Normandy and are very fresh! Eating oysters in Paris is very simple. At the bar *à huîtres* (oyster bar) and in restaurants, open oysters are served with lemon and shallot vinaigrette separately. I personally prefer to enjoy them plain. Our oysters are divided into two broad categories: the concave ones, which we call *creuses*, and the flat ones, called *plates*. The concave ones in particular come in different sizes (5 being the smallest and 0 the largest), flavors, and textures.

From north to south, we have seven regions dedicated to oyster farming: Normandy, northern Brittany, southern Brittany, Centre-Ouest, Marennes-Oléron, Arcachon, and the Mediterranean. Some of these regions are perhaps more famous than others, but they all produce excellent oysters. Oyster farming in the Mediterranean, especially

MY TIP
With oysters, I recommend a dry white wine like a Chardonnay. Personally, I love Saint-Véran, a Chardonnay from southern Burgundy. But if you absolutely want to eat oysters with red wine, then choose a simple red with just the right amount of acidity, like a Gamay de Touraine. A very Parisian address? *L'Huitrade* oyster bar at *Le Chiberta* restaurant. Top-quality oysters. A must! Just a stone's throw away from the Arc de Triomphe. See the Grand Huîtres (big oyster plate) signed by chefs Guy Savoy and Stéphane Laruelle.

in the Bassin de Thau, is rather specific, however it allows for the production of good-quality oysters, although they're less popular than the ones that come from the Atlantic coast. The French are experts and very demanding when it comes to the characteristics of the product. One thing's for sure, you're not going to see a genuine Parisian eating oysters that don't come from France.

Parenting

Are Parisian youngsters any calmer, more polite, or better behaved than other kids? Let me reassure you, they too get bad grades at school from time to time, don't really like to go to bed at night, and show the same artistic spirit (not always to our taste) when they make street art in their bedrooms. So when you see a young mom who is always impeccable, with model children, you might wonder what the secret is to French parenting.

Lou, an active and ravishing *Parisienne* in her 30s, finds time to do it all: work as a medical journalist, volunteer for charity, raise three young children with her CEO husband, and even race cars! Not to mention her involvement in what the media call the "Urban Green Market," when the city literally "turns green": boulevards, gardens, as well as roofs, balconies and building facades, become the ideal places for growing plants and flowers.

"How does this Parisian girl manage to keep looking cool and fresh at 7:00 P.M. in her little navy blue *Claudie Pierlot* dress, with her discreetly manicured nails? How does she manage to keep her kids spotless throughout the day? The little guys wear slim jeans *Bonton* and their little sister a *Petit Bateau* skirt and cardigan or a little black dress like her mom. Never, ever, will her kids be seen wearing loud colors, jogging trousers, or princess dresses. How does this young mother do it? She's constantly on the run but her kids are so nice and calm! Paris is a small-scale city for a capital of its importance. The sidewalks are narrow, the elevators are teensy, and the apartments are small, even if they're cozy and practical. Paris is just right for our little munchkins! They're at home in cramped little shops; they deftly squeeze through passengers' legs in crammed city buses. They proudly climb onto wooden horses on the city's old-fashioned carousels. As soon as they've finished their day at preschool, Jacques, Blanche, Scarlett, and Auguste rush to Parc Monceau, Jardin

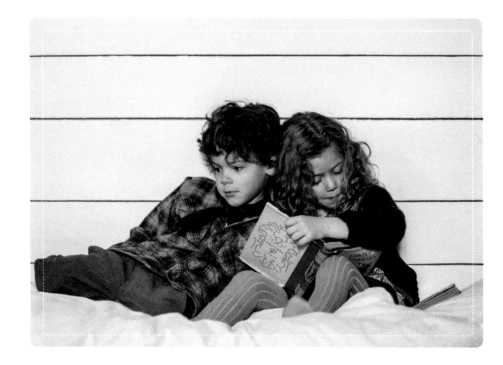

du Luxembourg, or another Parisian park. There they can run, jump, and climb under the watchful eye of their nanny. They practically never fight (ok, they do sometimes squabble a little). Good manners are *de rigueur*. They are taught to say hello, please, and thank you to everyone: 'Bonjour Madame,' 'S'il vous plaît Madame,' 'Merci Madame.' Children are used to going with their parents to neighborhood merchants such as the baker, who will spoil them with a little treat (even though they're too well brought up to ask for anything), or the cheese seller, who will have them try a fruity piece of Comté (Parisians start developing a refined palate early in life). Parisian life is human-scale. You can get around your neighborhood by *Vélib'*, the city bikes. It's a good place for kids to develop a social life, which is a must, even at a young age. Kids help carry veggies home from the organic food co-op and help to make the meal, learning to recognize fresh fruit and real garden vegetables. Traditionally, there's no school on Wednesdays here, so Parisian tykes stay home, learning to bake little French cakes like madeleines. There are never too many toys in his or her room—just a few carefully chosen playthings to avoid a mess and to help the little one concentrate on one game or toy at a time. The evening is often arts and crafts time, making collages or painting a page out of a children's magazine. No TV. The little guy or gal seems to fall asleep so much more easily after a bedtime story, and mom loves to read aloud the fairytales that her own mother used to read to her. So when do these mini-Parisians, who love museums, good food, and nice clothes, find time for shenanigans? A strict upbringing means rules, but rules are made to be broken. What a joy it is to hear stifled giggles coming from the next bedroom, where brother and sister, daubed with mom's makeup, are taking selfies with dad's tablet. Oh, well, sometimes you just have to let kids be kids. That's one of the secrets to living happily ever after in the city of the Tour Eiffel, the Louvre, and Notre-Dame."

Lou, Rue de Rome, January 15

LINKS
- Attitude
- Children
- Christmas
- Melancholy

Pastry Shops

Ahhhhh, Parisian pastry shops! Have you ever fallen into a swoon in front of one of those windows where the sweets in their holiday clothes seem to wink provocatively at you? It happens to me every day! Pastries—the Parisian's little sin! Yet when you ask the French which desserts are their favorites, it seems that their tastes are quite simple and traditional: dark chocolate cake takes first place followed by chocolate mousse, crêpes, *île flottante, tarte aux pommes,* and, in sixth place ... Italian tiramisu. While most of the time these daily pleasures are simple, the haute couture of the pastry world comprises *Saint-Honoré* by *Pierre Conticini, Opéra* by *Lenôtre,* and *Ispahan* by *Pierre Hermé.* Of the creations that are all the rage in the capital, sweets and desserts become real works of art, real luxuries, but ones that are affordable. In addition to the creations mentioned, pastry chefs often reinterpret the classic French pastries—*charlotte, fraisier, millefeuilles, tarte Tatin*—to give them a new look and a more current and personal flavor. Have you tried the *Paris-Brest* by *Jacques Genin? Ladurée* makes a pastry I just can't

LINKS
• Baguette
• Macaroons
• Madeleine

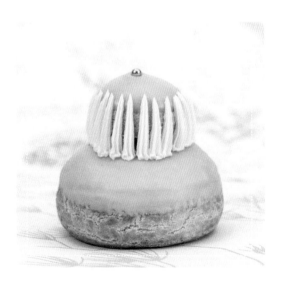

THE RECIPE
This is my childhood recipe. My mother would make it on a Sunday. Here's my suggestion for the perfect charlotte: avoid soaking the biscuits too much so they don't get soggy. The middle of the ladyfinger has to stay slightly hard so that the dessert will be firm. Arrange them so that they overlap slightly.

My mother's charlotte

Serves 4
14 ladyfingers
1 lb. 12 oz. peeled fresh pears or pears in syrup
1 1/2 cup sugar
1/2 vanilla bean
1 1/2 tbsp. butter for the mold
For the vanilla sauce
1 cup milk
3/4 cup granulated sugar
3 egg yolks
2 1/2 sheets of gelatin
1 vanilla bean
For the chantilly cream
1 cup crème fraîche (soured cream)
1/4 cup cold milk
1/8 cup "creamed" ice cream
1 tbsp. sugar
1 packet of vanilla-flavored powdered sugar
For the coulis
2 lbs. 3 oz. strawberries
1 1/2 cup sugar
1 tbsp. lemon juice

Use a brush dipped in melted butter to lightly grease the edges of a charlotte mold of 9 inches in diameter. Line the bottom with a disk of parchment paper. Dip the ladyfingers in a syrup made with water and sugar (or fruit liqueur) and arrange them along the sides, making sure they fit snugly and are even with the edge of the mold.

For the vanilla sauce: beat 3 egg yolks with 3/4 cup of sugar. Bring the milk to a boil with the vanilla bean. Add the milk to the beaten egg yolks, place over low heat and allow to thicken without boiling. Use a wooden spoon to stir. When warm fold in the gelatin sheets after soaking in water. Refrigerate.

For the chantilly cream: in a very cold bowl combine the crème frâiche, cold milk, 1 tablespoon of sugar, ice cream, and packet of powdered sugar. Use an electric mixer to beat for 6-8 minutes, then refrigerate the chantilly cream.

To cook the pears (if fresh), make a syrup with 2 cups of water, 1 1/2 cup of sugar and 1/2 vanilla bean. When the mixture starts boiling add the pears and cook until they're shiny. Drain the pears. Take 2/3 of the chantilly cream and delicately fold it into the vanilla sauce. Fill the mold alternating the sauce + chantilly cream and the pears. Refrigerate for at least 2 1/2 hours. Use the leftover chantilly cream to decorate the charlotte after removing it from the mold.

For the coulis: wash and cleanse the strawberries, whip them together with the lemon juice until you obtain a cream.

resist: a rose & raspberry *Religieuse* (photo). It's "to die for!" The contemporary Parisian pastry shop is a show of colors, shapes, and delicious details. The pastry chefs are artists in all respects, engaged in a continuous search for innovation and perfection in the flavors and textures that will make their desserts unique and magical. Now is the golden age of pastry in Paris, so let's take advantage of it, right? The creations of *Claire Damon*, especially the rhubarb *Chou* (puffs). All the sweets, without exception, by *Arnaud Larher* (*Meilleur Ouvrier de France* in 2007), a genius of taste and texture who knows how to surprise with both sophisticated creations and something simpler, like his almond *Pavé de Montmartre*—fab-u-lous! An address? The *Gâteaux Thoumieux* pastry shop. I love everything that chef *Jean-François Piège* does, but when he joins the pastry wizard *Ludovic Chaussard* to create sublime sweets without additives or preservatives, the result is extraordinary. My husband loves his *Tarte au citron* (lemon tart). The list of my favorites has to include *Christophe Adam*, the master of the éclair—fresh, delicious, and light ... in a word: modern. An address in the Marais, for gourmands "who watch their weight": *Les Fées Pâtissières* with incomparable mini reproductions of classic French pastries.

Perfume

Have you noticed that the word perfume begins with "P" like Paris? It is a wonderful subject that has inspired centuries of writers and filmmakers as well as the best "noses" of the world in search of THE fragrance that best represents Paris and the perfumes that most appeal to the Parisian woman. The result: a multitude of scented candles and fragrances inspired by the *Ville Lumière*. As for the *Parisienne*, the ideal perfume is the one that makes her dream, at times the one that best reflects her personality without excessively accentuating it, but always the invisible accessory that completes her look—the olfactory signature that she leaves in her wake.

• The scent of the Parisian woman. Whether she is discrete, feminine, extroverted, sensitive, seductive, uninhibited, or a dreamer, each Parisian wears her own perfume. Sometimes it takes years before she finds the perfect fragrance, the one that represents her character, emotions, and style. There's the Parisian woman who is looking for a brand new fragrance, the rare essence that no one else wears, and the one who selects her perfume for the dreamy content of its commercials and publicity photos, a great love story, or an erotic fairytale moment, and for the message that it emanates—"sexy but refined," "classy but authentic," "always on the go but beautiful." Then there are lightning strikes that can last a lifetime or vanish in a moment. My friend Astride's love story with perfumes is very typical:

LINKS
• Femininity
• Makeup
• Seduction

"I have worn *Diorissimo* since I was thirteen years old—an incredible find. A perfume masterpiece created by Christian Dior in 1956. I happened to not wear it

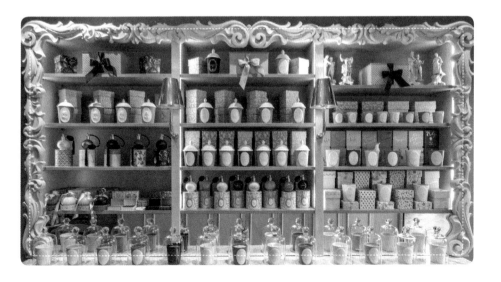

one summer and when, in September, I found myself
immersed in a cloud of just collected lily of the valley,
I was dancing and spinning with joy. A few years ago,
on holiday in Florida, I entered a large department store
in Palm Beach and was captured by a scent. Excited,
curious, almost obsessed with finding the object of this
sudden passion, I can still see myself sniffing like a fox
terrier searching for the beloved fragrance: *Déclaration
de Cartier.* A wonderful scent, but the romance lasted only
one summer! This olfactory excitement came over me
again as I passed the Creed store in London. A woman
coming out left behind her a strange hint of amber and
orange blossom, a very refined and delicate mixture
that immediately transported me into a state of ecstasy.
Closing my eyes, notes of incense started to penetrate
me ... I entered the store. This sweet but dry perfume is
called *Angelique Encens.* Today it is no longer produced,
but since that day, I call it the 'scent of the unknown' in
memory of the woman who unknowingly introduced
me to it. I always have it with me, a powerful scent, for
my 'femme fatale' moments. Olivier Creed created it for
Marlene Dietrich, an actress I love!"

The Parisian woman believes in the power of her perfume.
It is a presence, a love story made to last, and that's why
she loves beautiful perfumes that are able to give her
thrills and happiness at every reunion.
• The scent of Paris. I don't think you can sum up Paris
in one smell. In his book *Perfume,* Patrick Suskind
describes the smells of an *Ancien Régime* Paris that
no longer exists; my friend Marc from Boston speaks
to me of the odors of seafood stalls, of macaroons, and
many other wonders that arouse his olfactory memory.
Even those memoires that come more spontaneously to
the mind are quite "sweet": the smell of freshly baked
bread and croissants, of the crêpes sold in small kiosks of
old Paris. Then I think of "Paris in the rain" and the smell
of earth mixed with salt on wet stone—very characteristic,

MY TIP

I won't list all the great creators of fragrances that can be found only in Paris for fear of forgetting someone. I love all the beautiful authentic and rare perfumes, and when my olfactory curiosity stimulates me, I go to one of the places dedicated to rare and precious perfumes like *Jovoy* in the 1st arrondissement or *Nose* in the 2nd. *Le Bon Marché Rive Gauche* is great for fragrance shopping. The new website 24sevres.com has a fantastic catalog of perfumes. The only problem is that you cannot try them online. (Maybe one day?) A marvelous spot worth visiting for fragrances, teas, and scented candles is the new Ladurée boutique on Rue de Rivoli, a tiny, very Parisian boudoir.

especially in summer when a thunderstorm violently bathes the hot cobblestones. I love Place Dauphine in the spring, when the scent of the chestnut trees in bloom is combined with that of the sand and old stones. There are many perfumers and creators of scented candles searching for the magic recipe that most faithfully represents the city. For some, Paris is above all "plants." They recall the scent of lilies in luxury shops, of the sumptuous flowers that *Jeff Leatham* puts out every day at the Four Seasons George V Hotel, of the ivy that cascades down the facades of buildings, and of the flowers that adorn the balconies. For others, Paris is a very pronounced odor of wood and wax that one smells climbing the stairs of old buildings, or that of the parquet, wainscoting, and antiques of old apartments, so faithfully interpreted in the *Bois Précieux* candle by *Rigaud*. Another is the scent of wood and beeswax—that of the stages of Paris theaters and of the *Opéra* candle from *Astier de Villatte*. *Solis*, the candle from the house of *Trudon*, transports us to the *Galerie des Glaces* (Hall of Mirrors) of the Palace of Versailles. The *Rue Saint-Victor* candle reveals the scent of old books characteristic of antiquarian booksellers. For *Inès de la Fressange*, the smell of the capital and of her candle *Week-end à Paris* is the smell of the Parisian woman's leather handbag and her lipstick. The pastry shop *Ladurée* took inspiration from the luxurious fragrance of tuberose to create its *Paris* candle. For me, the smell which evokes Paris is the one you discover on entering a Parisian's home: a mix of hardwood floors and white flowers, just like that of *Maison*, Sophie the Parisian's parfume.

Plastic Surgery

A tricky subject to bring up in Paris, where no one admits anything! On one hand, there are magazines and clinics vaunting the benefits of plastic surgery; on the other, there's the section of the Parisian intelligentsia who, out of tradition and education, scorn the cult of the body and artificial changes to what Mother Nature gave us. Plastic surgery raises an obvious problem in society: women, but also men, are being increasingly influenced by physical appearance to the point of basing their social relations and relationships on the visual message it delivers. Hence the generalization regarding plastic surgery. In general, the Parisian hates ostentation, whether it relates to her bust, her makeup, or the length of her skirt; she questions everything in order to avoid what she considers social

MY TIP
Don't forget that seduction in Paris is a subtle game of a gradual revelation, not showing everything you've got all at once, and part of the work of a good surgeon comes from understanding the relationship his patient has between her physique and seduction.

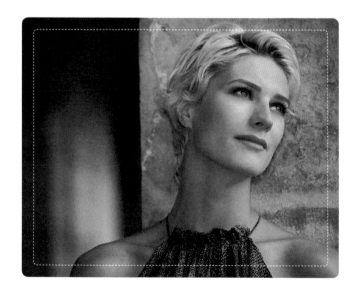

"death": being classed as tasteless! Plastic surgery is one of her demons because it goes against her "I do or I don't," "if you can see it, what would I look like" education. Whether the motivation is to feel better about herself or to correct whatever body part she wants to improve, the Parisian woman takes an ultra-moderate, subtle approach and will only pick a surgeon who shares her views. Well informed, she knows that excessive surgery creates the opposite effect and makes you look older in the majority of cases, as she's seen with many film stars. As for over-plump lips, she doesn't think it's natural or sexy—it's just "plain bad taste!"

"French men don't like big breasts," said a Parisian surgeon whose reputation is partly due to his moderation. "The Parisian woman likes just the right amount, a bit of a boost for her bust but without making her companion's jaw drop."

Among the trends of great French actresses and Parisian women, the most popular are breast implants and face and eyelid lifts.

"We live in a society where youth ... is considered the most valuable asset ... We know very well that no cosmetic surgery or even the most effective wrinkle creams will make us feel younger or more healthy. The secret of a long life and good health is within our body. I call this new medical approach that acts on the origin of aging internal cosmetic surgery."

Hervé Grosgogeat, a nutritionist specialized in biology and sports medicine (author of many publications), Paris

Plating

In Paris, when you judge a dish, even if taste comes first, plating is also primordial. When food is presented attractively on the plate, it whets the appetite.

The Parisian woman is conditioned to notice the visual

aspect of the food she eats or serves. The presentation must be pretty but not too complicated, so that it shows off the chef's talent. The concept is that, with a little skill, any food can become a visual delight, even a rare rib of beef or plain old mayonnaise. What's more, with French *nouvelle cuisine,* dating back to the 1970s, gravies no longer contain starch. The modern trend focuses more on natural cooking juices, which actually look nicer on the plate.

• Take a good look at your ingredients and think about how you are going to arrange them on the plate. Work with shape, cut, and color to bring out the interior beauty of each product. Fresh seasonal vegetables are the fashion these days. The way they look on the plate is important.

• Be nonconformist. Dare to mix styles. Wasabi, herbs, and spices can vary the colors and textures of your dish.

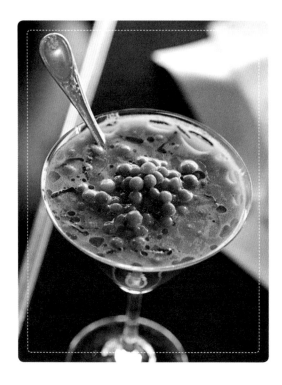

MY TIP
• Choose simple-looking tableware. The plate shouldn't steal the show from what's on it. What you want guests to remember is how good your food was, not how colorful your plates looked, so choose pure and simple designs like square white plates for meat in brown gravy, or transparent tableware for salads in order to bring out the different colors of the ingredients. You can find fantastic plates at *Geneviève Lethu* and *Christofle* and less expensive ones at *La Vaissellerie* and *Porcelaine Blanche*.
• Add gravy at the last moment at the dinner table. In today's French cooking, sauce is often considered a condiment rather than a main ingredient, so serve it accordingly. You can always put a little bit of sauce on each plate and then invite guests to serve themselves if they want more, or ceremoniously pass around an attractive gravy boat.

• Add the most colorful ingredients last to enliven the plate and create depth.
• Create an "unstructured" look. It's modern to present traditional dishes and make them look trendy. For example, lay your basic vegetables on the bottom of the plate then add other foods according to color, keeping the main food clearly in sight.
• Consider a "monochromatic" theme. For example, "white on white," which is actually fairly easy to do in cooking. You can contrast different shades of white and different textures by combining foods such as asparagus and scallops, or white meat and potatoes in the same dish.
• Serve the food hot. That means staying away from time-consuming presentations when you have more than four dinner guests. In that case, limit it to just three attractively presented dishes.
• Find an original way to serve one of the ingredients and put it on top of the plate. For example, beet chips or a scoop of parsley ice cream!

Polka dots

My friend Susan from Seattle thinks that polka dots are the perfect symbol of French elegance! Without a doubt, because they are an eternal wink to the 1960s, and are in

MY TIP
Warning, polka dots are not always easy to wear. So as not to overdo it, limit their use to the top or bottom, to be combined with a basic article of your wardrobe.

fact a milestone in fashion, polka dots are always valid, especially in Paris. Casual, classic or trendy, they are revisited in every new season, in a mini or maxi version, in a total look or in small doses. Fashion and polka dots, a love story that lasts over time, with ups and downs. This year, polka dots have landed in all-over collections, graphics, 3D, black and white: in short, they are ubiquitous and appear to be "almost" indispensable!

• Blue sweater with a 1950s polka-dot skirt + a large men's watch + trench coat + oversized glasses.

• White cigarette pants + polka-dot blouse + narrow waist jacket + moccasins.

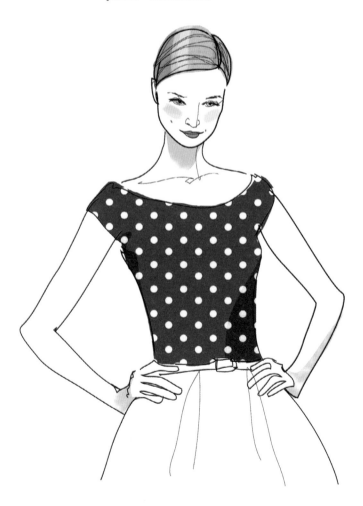

HISTORY
In the 1930s, polka dots had their apogee in the fashion world. Printed on muslin or silk and in various colors, they were adored by seamstresses and women in general. With Pop Art in the 1960s—particularly the paintings of Roy Lichtenstein—they were revamped and became trendy again.

For the Parisian woman, fashion shows are only a source of inspiration, a way "to keep up with the trends," but the real creation happens when she is in front of her closet and her neurons combine basic pieces + fashion articles + accessories to have a "fashionable but free Parisian" look. Yes to polka dots, but no to a "Minnie" (Mickey Mouse's girlfriend) or retro pin-up look.

R

Rain

If I told you that it doesn't rain that much in Paris, would you believe me? But it's true, if we compare the number of rainy days in the French capital to the number in other major Western cities, we are far from the top. The weather is gray and cloudy rather than wet. I acknowledge that I have also noticed that it rains more on weekends than during the week! It seems to be an effect of pollution. In any case, you must admit that Paris has its charm, even in the rain. Especially at night, the lights on wet streets and sidewalks are truly magical. A nice romantic walk under a huge umbrella in the lanes of the Île Saint-Louis is an unforgettable experience, don't you think? Have you ever seen the Place de la Concorde in the rain or the Pont Alexandre III with its *Horses of Marly* and the Grand Palais in the background? On the other hand, it is also true that, for both the Parisian and the tourist, rain during the day is not much fun—not for getting around, clothing, or hairstyles. It's difficult to stay glamorous and smiling under a winter downpour. Although we hate the rain combined with terrible gusts of wind, a light drizzle does not interfere with our lives—maybe it ruins our mood, but

LINKS
• Grayness
• Melancholy
• Sky

MY TIP
My three must-have items for rainy days: black rubber *Aigle* boots (functional but also suitable for a urban look), an elegant black rain hat from *Maison Michel*, a super-light mini umbrella from *Isotoner*, and of course, my go-everywhere black trench coat! What more do I need? A smile, because I hate rain!

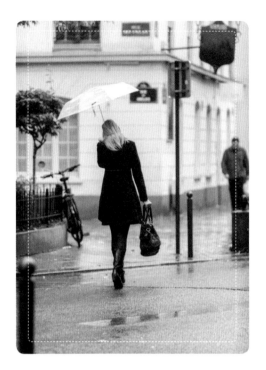

we both have plenty to do! In addition to the great classic rainy trips, museums, exhibitions, and department stores, you can visit the tropical aquarium of the Porte Dorée, browse at *Deyrolle* (the temple of taxidermy), or roam the streets and galleries of the Belle Epoque. If none of these appeals to you, there is always a good cup of hot chocolate in a tearoom or a tour of pastry shops searching for the best *millefeuille* in the capital! What is it that the Parisian woman fears the most? Short winter days + a lead gray sky + rain + a temperature of 30°F!

Red

Unbelievable ... only in Paris could the supremacy of the legendary little black dress start to give way to the glamour of red. Of course there's red and there's red (fifty shades of red?!), but only the right red will do. The *Parisienne* speaks of a "Saint-Laurent red" when she marries it with fuchsia, and a "Chanel red" for a classic shade of nail polish. *Rouge criard* means "loud red" like the color of her coworker's car, and *rouge pouffiasse,* or "bitchy red," applies to trashy or slutty apparel, especially if over-accessorized. *Rouge petard* is a flashy red like Ferrari red. "Ultra-red" means whatever shade of red is in vogue. Finally, the Parisian uses the phrase *un beau rouge* to mean the exact shade of red she happens to think is perfect—for her long dress, nail polish, or cashmere sweater. She is a perfectionist by nature, knows how to recognize the perfect red out of one thousand hues. She knows how to wear it with moderation to stay elegant, and she knows a multitude of ways for adding just the right

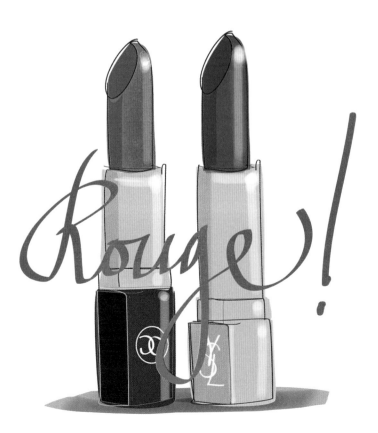

touch of red to her outfit: a coat, a handbag, a sexy dress, or a pair of gloves. In winter she livens up her everyday look by adding red accents to more conservative colors: sometimes black, but mostly gray, beige, or even white. A red belt with a man's jacket or white jeans can be the little detail that brightens up the outfit and makes it chic. Red lace lingerie, especially for blondes! *Simone Pérèle, Aubade,* or *Etam*—the Parisian loves classic French brands that "flaunt her stuff" with elegance. It's glamorous under a denim shirt, a *Petit Bateau marinière,* or an *Agnès B* smart casual jacket. A little detail of Parisian seduction: let a little red lace "accidentally show on purpose" under an *Eric Bombard* v-neck cashmere sweater.

As for sweaters, nothing frilly or hand-knit if you want to look chic. Chose a big red *Givenchy, Isabel Marant,* or *Carol* sweater with slim white, black, or gray pants or a pencil skirt. A little red sweater is *magnifique* with a white blouse, a quality black leather skirt, and black heels (red stimulates the endocrine glands, which increase adrenalin levels, which in turn can lead to animal urges, so a pair of four-inch *Louboutin* just might be overkill). A symbol of sensuality, warmth, and fire, red is the color to wear for a date. However, it's not an easy color for all women to wear, since it denotes an outgoing personality. Wearing a red dress to a dinner implies the woman won't mind being the center of attention. If you are normally shy or reserved, wearing red can either boost your self-confidence or have the opposite effect and make you feel too self-conscious. Before you buy a red *Hervé Léger* dress, make sure you're capable of wearing it. I wore a long red dress on my wedding day!

Rive Gauche, Rive Droite

Seen from the other side of the Atlantic, there is only one type of *Parisienne* associated with inhabitants of *La Ville Lumière* in general. But seen from the inside, things are very different. There are many types of Parisian women, depending on education, family situation, and social class. But, in the end, they can be divided into two categories: *Miss Rive Gauche* and *Miss Rive Droite* (Left Bank or Right Bank of the Seine). Worthy representatives of two distinct areas that, like in a boxing match, compete for the title of Paris with a capital "P": the modern Paris of the Right Bank—that of the Champs-Elysées, Avenue Montaigne, and Place Vendôme; and the Paris of the Left Bank—the Latin Quarter, Lutèce, and Saint-Germain-des-Prés. If Parisians are allies in being hated by the rest of France, particularly by the south, they will dismember one another when it comes to determining who has more monuments and churches and especially who owns the soul and mind

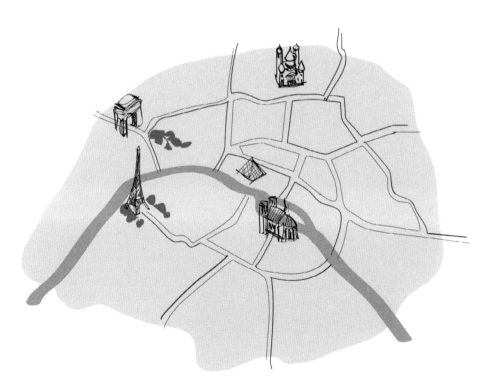

of Paris. Since this is the crux of the problem, the Rive Gauche woman—intellectual and elitist, haughty and proud of her membership in that club—considers the Rive Droite woman to be shallow, vulgar in her display of luxury. The latter—aristocratic, modern, and dynamic—considers the Rive Gauche woman to be an antiquated snob. In both quarters, there is no lack of arguments to unfairly tear up the opponent.

Even celebrities choose their bank of the Seine based on its spirit: there are the stars of the Marais, the Palais-Royal, the Triangle d'Or, the Rue Saint-Honoré, and the Trocadéro (Right Bank), and those of Saint-Sulpice, the Île Saint-Louis, and the Jardin du Luxembourg, who like to breathe the same air as Beauvoir, Gide, Juliette Greco, Hemingway, Sartre, and Serge Gainsbourg—all the celebrities who created the legend of Saint-Germain-des-Prés and the intellectual but chic Left Bank *parisianisme*. Paris is a city on a human scale. If every quarter claims its own identity and its local urban folklore, the sense of belonging to a bank is strong. The Rive Droite certainly has ways of dressing that are a bit more "casual chic," while the elegance of the Rive Gauche is a bit more fashion. But beware: paradoxically, there is only one Parisian woman because, if the Rive Droite has its Bastille Day and the Rive Gauche its revolution of May 1968, the two banks form a united front against the world when it comes to demonstrating for freedom, as happened in January 2015. Is it the strength of Paris's bridges that unites us?

Roofs

The roofs of Paris are symbols of the capital, a favorite theme of photographers, painters, and poets. They often have little balconies in the garrets, gardens, or terraces where the Parisian woman loves to dream, write in her diary, or relax with a coffee. Barbara came to Paris thirty years ago. Born in Italy, she became a true Parisian girl, the perfet combination of elegance, bohème, and naturalness. A svelte and sophisticated woman, one that, with a sudden laughter, switches from solemnity to lightness! She is passionate about the French *art de vivre*, and the *Ville Lumière* continues to fascinate her and energize her every day. I just adore the way she describes her "love affair" with Parisian roofs: "I love Paris in all seasons! But mostly Paris roofs in the autumn. I like to look out the window of my fifth-floor bedroom. There is a very nice perspective of cascading roofs opening up in front of my eyes, just like when, as a child, I used to stare at the Nativity scene: a sort of enchanted stupor. When the weather is nice, I can sit on my balcony in the sun and simply contemplate the roofs and chimneys of the city. The morning sunlight reflects on the tin roofs like a smooth caress, I can see some smoke coming out of a chimney, I imagine a nice couple playing with each other's hands, sipping some Bordeaux wine while listening to Gainsbourg's *La Javanaise* ... I can see a window slightly open with some shirts hanging outside, giving some color to the city and movement like Calder's mobiles. Now there is a cat's silhouette inside the other window moving its tail in a nonchalant way, just like

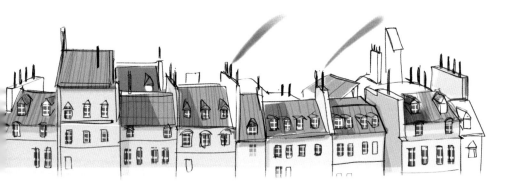

O'Malley from *The Aristocats* movie. How funny to see a small wild plant coming out of another chimney—must have been some seed that found a cozy nest to give birth. Lucky plant! It can see even a better view than I from up there! What a sky today!"
Barbara, Rue des Batignolles, February 11

S

Sales

The Parisian has a hyper-rational way to shop at sales. Although she loves the big names, in particular for the basics of her wardrobe, she wouldn't even dream of paying full price! Special discounts for the press, staff discounts through her "best girlfriend," outlets, pre-sales, private sales, and official sales—all are good for smart shopping at more affordable prices. This is an art that she controls well, knowing the risks: buying a useless article, the wrong dress, the one that will quickly go out of style, and the one that is too expensive despite the lower price; going and coming home empty-handed or knocking yourself for mediocre results, trying to give your wardrobe a breath of fresh air and filling it with duplicates ... And the worst thing for a Parisian woman is buying in quantity at the expense of quality! Having learned from her negative experiences, she adopts a well-established and unbeatable strategy.

• She starts seriously planning for sales several days in advance, in front of her closet, armed with pen and paper. "What do I need (my basics), what do I want (a bit more fashion or color), what labels do I like to wear, which accessories can I buy to give my look a shot in the arm, which pants and skirts need a top and vice versa?" This is a moment of self-criticism about purchases made at the latest sales and never worn! She makes a good shopping list, puts limits on her budget, and lists the mistakes to avoid in black and white, the seasonal color that she adores but that he doesn't like at all, the silk clothing she

MY TIP
In Paris, winter sales begin on the second Wednesday of January and summer sales on the last Wednesday of June for a period of six weeks! So it's easy to plan your trip and your budget! For more information, visit the website of the Paris Tourism Office.

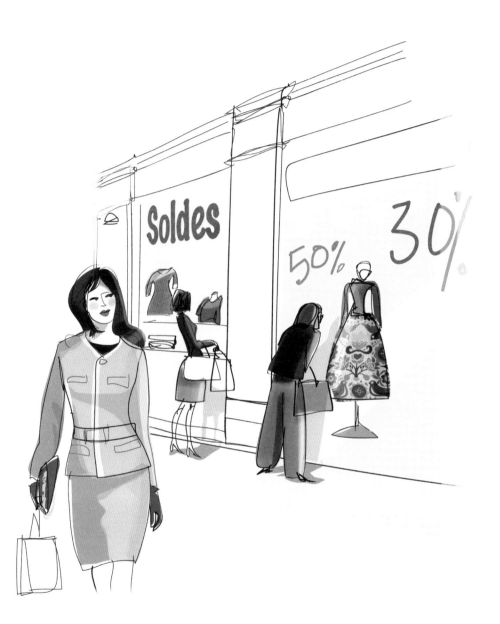

hates ironing, and the styles she would love to wear but that he doesn't like. In short, like a professional buyer by trade, she sets limits on her mission.

• With her short list and possibly some clothes to match, she begins a tour of the stores a few days before, at lunchtime or between appointments, to stake out her hunting grounds, where she can satisfy her desires, find her necessities, and her "loves at first sight." She will take advantage of the opportunity to try on things that will leave salesgirls disappointed and ask if she can come back on the eve of the sale. It costs nothing to ask, right?

• Go to a sale when everyone else does? No way! The Parisian knows the right time to make her rounds far from the crowd: the first day or the last day for opportunities during the week; in the morning, when the store opens; and absolutely never on Saturday and not even at 6:00 P.M., when twenty-five women are fighting over the last blue sweater, which isn't anything special anyway.

• The Parisian is elegant but practical. She will adapt her look to the task of the day with an outfit that is chic but suitable for trying on clothes. She will leave the high heels at home and opt for a pair of black ballerinas, ideal for trying on everything; she will wear a skirt instead of pants, which is more practical for waiting in line for a dressing room; she will carry a shoulder bag to keep her hands free; and "appropriate" underwear (even if single, she almost always wears appropriate underwear, because she loves to pamper herself starting with what she's got on underneath).

• Even in the heat of the moment, the Parisian woman is able to remain lucid. She came for a sale and will not tear out her hair for the new collection; she comes to shop for three hours and has no intention of spending the whole day or coming back again. However, she has a budget that she cannot go over, and, like all women, she will exceed it. She plans to buy only basic items but she will let herself be tempted by the must-have fashion accessories of the season!

Seduction

What a dangerous and difficult subject! I can't reveal too much or my girlfriends will lynch me, and I have to be careful not to fall into clichés, but three things are certain, official, and admissible about the Parisian woman and seduction: her seductiveness is not only physical; she puts her whole self into it, as with everything she does; she grants her favors only with an eyedropper!

• In Paris you don't have to be 5'8", have a thirty-seven-inch bust, and a model's legs to conquer a man! Humor, spirit, confidence, and unpredictability are also important cards in the game of seduction. They are the trump cards that allow her to attract, but also to consolidate, her nascent relationship. Nothing is taken for granted in a market where more and more women are seeking a soul

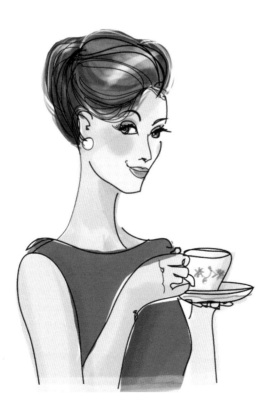

MY TIP
Why not work on your voice, humor, conversation, or empathy rather than resorting systematically and exclusively to Botox and scalpels? And this, among other things, is what Madame Claude's call-girls learn: how to seduce and be liked by their clients. "The important thing is the other person," said the famous *maîtresse*. In other words: take an interest in what the guy likes in order to get his attention and understand his emotions. And remember that it is better, and sexier in the long run, to fall in love with a caring, funny, and/or cultured man than with a dandy who thinks only about parties with friends: I've heard that the epitome of snobbery these days is to claim that you are "sapiosexual"!

mate. In Paris, where bling-bling seduction is considered vulgar, the heavy artillery—namely, charm, freshness, and interesting conversation—is much more effective than "wiggling your butt" on five-inch *Louboutin* heels or a neckline that plunges to your navel. So before you go to a plastic surgeon to remake what nature gave you from A to Z, carefully consider if it will really change anything. A Parisian who doesn't have a "perfect" figure is well aware that she also has a chance by making good use of her arsenal of seduction: charisma, kindness (which, by the way, is very trendy these days), talent, and the ability to listen (the queen of hearts of the game). Pay attention: even beautiful women can use these cards instead of following seduction manuals that say the opposite on the assumption that men only fall in love with women who play hard to get—a method that may work at first, but that is tiresome in the long run, especially in Paris! The Parisian woman has made a habit, since she was a little girl, of cultivating her own inner world and, over the years, using her charisma to seduce. It's a question of education rather than DNA, so everyone can do it.
• Be warned: the Parisian is highly motivated and dedicated, but that doesn't mean she's "easy." The famous *Voulez-vous coucher avec moi?* is almost always answered with a laugh or a slap but rarely succeeds. The Parisian seduction technique is similar to whipping egg whites. Our mothers have told us a thousand times: "To make a good soufflé or chocolate mousse, you have to beat the

egg whites slowly until they become beautifully firm."
In Paris this is the whole trick: we like "slow seduction"
to create "enduring desire." We cultivate mystery and
silence rather than blabbing information. Small doses
arouse curiosity and a desire to know more the next
time! We reveal our inner sensuality very slowly by
sending encrypted messages. And the Parisian woman's
official strategy is a skillful mix of unpredictability and
enchantment. According to the film *French Kiss*, "The
Parisian woman thinks 'yes' but says 'no' and vice versa."
We switch from ice cold to warm and tender or from
indifference to interest (and vice versa) in an instant,
which forces the other person to pay more attention
and make a more consistent effort—while we are sending
sensual messages with naked shoulders, glimpsed,
of course, under a low-cut sweater with a lovely bra strap
that appears innocently when we take off our jacket; with
immaculately groomed feet that prance in delightful
sandals; with a skirt that lifts slightly when we sit
at the table of a bistro; with a glimpse of lingerie under
a silk blouse; with that cowlick of hair that breaks away
from the bun and that never stops swinging between her
ear and the corner of her lips. And yes, uncovering your
body does not mean being sexy. A Parisian would say that
a too-deep neckline, too-short skirt, and uncovered navel
are "simply ugly"!

See-through

A few days ago, I was doing a "spot of shopping" in Paris
with my Italian friend Margherita. We were wandering
around the Place des Victoires district looking for some
fab "typically Parisian" outfits for her. I took her to *Kabuki*,
one of my favorite stores, to see the new collections and
renew my stock of *Equipment* blouses (this mythical brand
of 1990s fashion lovers is a key basic of the Parisian's
current wardrobe). While she was looking at the new

LINKS
• Accessories
• Basic Wear
• Vintage
• Wardrobe

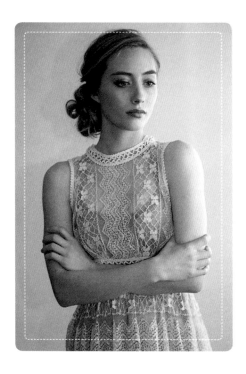

arrivals at *Givenchy* and *Balenciaga*, I tried on a pastel silk blouse; it was so feminine, so Parisian. I love these blouses; I've got them in a variety of colors and wear them all the time with skinny jeans or leather leggings. They are fantastic for an elegant glamorous-meets-androgynous look, "fashionably correct," and just sexy enough because my dark lace *Chantal Thomass* bra shows through lightly. I "generously" insisted that Margherita should get one too (generally, the Parisian woman hates one of her friends having the same garment as she, but between Rome and Paris the chances of us bumping into each other wearing exactly the same thing were low). Her response was surprising: "No, no, no, I couldn't wear a see-through blouse like that, it's indecent." Amazing. I explained to her the benefits of the Parisian woman's theory on seduction and sensuality: "Give them a hint but don't show too much." But I couldn't convince her. *Va bene*, I told her!

As we continued our trip, it was her turn to go into the fitting room and, to my great surprise, she ended up buying a red sweater: it was lovely but had such a low neckline you could see half of her size 36Bs! I couldn't help saying what I thought: "How can you wear that? I wouldn't dare!" For us Parisian women, the décolleté is a delicate subject; we always want to guard against being tasteless or showing off too much of our assets.

Shoes

In Paris, shoe stores compete in number with *pâtisseries*; there are more than fifteen of them in the Rue de Grenelle and Rue du Cherche-Midi alone! And for good reason, since the Parisian absolutely worships shoes and buys a lot of them. You can't deny the figures; we're massive consumers of shoes! The three real questions the *Parisienne* asks herself outside a shoe store are:
1. Shall I go for it?
2. More heels?
3. More black?
And then ...
1. She gives in—the time for therapy and a guilty conscience is long past!
2. We've got the reputation of being perched on heels twenty-four hours a day, which is a slight exaggeration. Although we adore heels and how feminine they make us feel, we don't go running in stilettos. But things have been changing recently, much to the dismay of podiatrists who won't have as many damaged feet to look after: flat shoes have entered the arena and are trying to steal the limelight from heels. In one camp are the chic fashion editors and fashion bloggers, and in the other, coquettes, lovers of traditional femininity and, of course, men. Are Parisian women going to give up glamour for comfort?
3. Observing Paris from a satellite, we see a mass of black centipedes that are none other than Parisian women's

LINKS
• Basic Wear
• Heels
• Little Black Dress
• Wardrobe

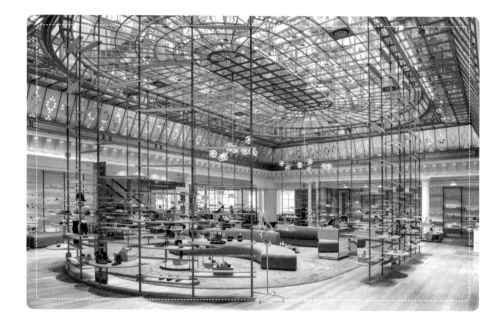

shoes! Mainly pumps, ballet flats, and boots. But, as always, the trend here is for change. Since the latest runway shows and, above all, since Inès de la Fressange launched her new patterned and colorful ballet flats, the Parisian is going for it and treading a new path with her choices.

The Parisian woman's basics:
• Ballerinas (ballet flats). Every year, fashion magazines tell us they're in or out, but looking at Parisians in the street, you'd think they were legally mandatory—they're everywhere. The ballet flat, first worn by Brigitte Bardot in the 1960s, is a timeless classic, the casual version of the pump.
• Pumps. We just adore them! They're great for all situations, go with everything, and slim the leg. This is THE favored shoe of the Parisian women, the one that occupies her heart and most of her closet!
• Chelsea and combat boots are still all the rage in Paris;

they're comfortable and practical, with a rock chic style. But how can we look sophisticated and feminine in them without looking like we're about to go horseback riding, a look that doesn't go down well with our loved one? According to all the "serious" surveys, Parisian men frankly don't like them and much prefer "girly" shoes or, on the other hand, *Dita Von Teese* stilettos. Whether they're heeled or flat, these boots must be good quality, in a dark color, and not too tight on the calf to have half a chance of getting into the manual of elegance.

• Knee high boots. Nothing better has ever been invented for stylishly keeping warm in the winter in Paris! With slim pants, a little dress, or a short skirt, the Parisian woman is never without them for a chic classy look. Even rubber boots have found their way from country life to city chic. *Aigle* boots are now the trendiest footwear on rainy Parisian streets. Mine are red to brighten up cloudy days.

• Sneakers. A mystery in the capital of style! Much criticized by the Parisian women who only swore by high heels, they've really come to the fore now. Even luxury couture houses are into them; *Chanel* sneakers have become something to dream about. Sneakers and figure-hugging black sweater dresses are seen in the best cafés in Paris. And once again, the Parisian has her own way of wearing them and still looking stylish. The secret: the sneakers are the only "sportswear" element of the look.

• Flat sandals are ultra-feminine and groomed feet are so sexy! The Parisian loves them; with a little dress or wide pants, she wears them with pride, leaving the heels at home but still looking glamorous and chic. Here again, it's all about contrasts; jeweled sandals with rolled up jeans, or leather pants or plain-woven sandals with a short or above-the-knee little dress. It's a question of age and legs.

• Heeled sandals. Even in winter, they're the best! My trick is to wear them with fine striped or flowery socks—my signature with a classic pant.

• We also love our brogues and loafers. We'd need more than a book to describe our passion for shoes.

Shopping Tour

Place des Victoires in the 1st arrondissement is one of the city's classic shopping spots. It's there we find our Parisian, with her best friend on her arm or her darling in tow, picking out the latest French fashions with simple but sophisticated good taste: oh-so-Parisian clothes, jewels, and accessories. It's also a good part of Paris to go shopping for household linens, home decoration ideas, and gifts (but Place des Victoires is not the only great shopping spot in town). Join me for a guided five-hour shopping tour. We'll start at 10:00 A.M. at the Etienne Marcel metro station, break for lunch at a nice bistro at Place des Victoires, and finish our day with a glass of fine wine at a wine merchant in the Galerie Vivienne, a nineteenth-century shopping arcade. Don't forget the concept: the Parisian is an independent and multifaceted shopper. She is trendy but never a fashion victim.

• Exit the metro onto Rue Etienne Marcel. At No. 15 Rue Etienne Marcel, have a look at *Declercq*, an extravaganza of home trimmings, fabrics, and decoration. Our fashion tour commences at No. 21, at *Ba&sh*, a brand created by girlfriends looking to put together the "ideal wardrobe." Everything there is ultra-feminine, modern, and incredibly Parisian. A few doors down, at No. 25, we find *Kabuki*, THE fashionista's boutique, with a nice collection of sublime designer clothes by the likes of *Alexander Wang*, *Balenciaga*, *Balmain*, *Barbara Bui*, *Givenchy*, *Kenzo*, and *Stella McCartney*, not to mention *Shourouk* jewelry. Next stop is *Naf Naf* at No. 33 for a fresh, young, impertinent style—nothing old-lady-like. Let's move on to *Comptoir des Cotonniers* at No. 35. You'll just love this brand's elegant city-girl style of easy-to-wear clothes for mother and daughter.

Now let's hop across the street to No. 42, where we find *Sandro*, the up-and-coming name in the world of premium ready-to-wear for the Parisian looking for a style that's more rock 'n' roll than *Comptoir des Cotonniers*, more

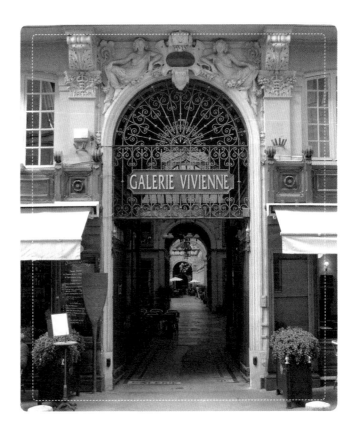

with-it than *Vanessa Bruno*, and more colorful than
Les Petites. At No. 44 reigns *The Kooples*, a rising star
in Paris. This French brand has a unique concept: "*The
Kooples* dresses Couples" (i.e., they feature coordinated
unisex style clothes for you and your beloved). At the
same spot, don't miss the multi-brand shop *By Marie* that
showcases both emerging and established designers. They
have vintage items as well as all sorts of things to strike
your fancy. Next stop, *Iro* at No. 46—a textbook case
of a brand that started off with pretty basic stuff but finally
took flight and is now the princess of Parisian street-style,
with apparel that is cool and glamorous. Now for a real
must: a visit to *Claudie Pierlot* at No. 49. Allow yourself
plenty of time to try things on, and you're sure to leave the

shop laden with shopping bags. Everything is tops there. Timeless styles distinguished by all kinds of little details to discretely catch a man's eye. Time to walk over to Place des Victoires. On the way, we'll stop off at *La Piscine*. This *piscine* is not a swimming pool, as its name suggests, but a 3,000-square-foot clearance outlet with bargains on brand name clothes. Once again, allow yourself plenty of time to browse.

• Our Parisian shopping odyssey continues with the shops at Place des Victoires, a circular plaza that owes its name to the victories of King Louis XIV (represented by the equestrian monument in the center of the square). Our next destination is *Apostrophe,* at No. 1 Place des Victoires, which features "second skin" clothing, with nice materials and pure simple cuts that will please active, sophisticated women who hate ostentation. *Apostrophe* is popular with French television celebrities and international politicians. (Let's do lunch ... I'll drop a few names.) If you appreciate really fine linens, check out *Yves Delorme* next door. Then at No. 2 we step into *Zadig & Voltaire*, one of the ultra-coolest brands on the planet. They've just modernized their Parisian line with some "basic" outfits that rock! On to No. 3 Place des Victoires, where we find *Gérard Darel*, a leading name in Paris for more than forty years. *Gérard Darel*'s unique vision of fashion is often inspired by iconic figures such as Jackie Kennedy and Marilyn Monroe. The styles of the 1950s are revisited with a modern twist. Next, if you love fashion jewelry, stop at *Agatha*, at No. 5—bracelets, rings, necklaces, earrings, and anklets galore. The style is lovely, fresh, and unpretentious. At the same address, *Les Petites* is another must. The look is a savvy blend of ethnic, vintage, and sensual romanticism (embroidery, lace, and delicate materials). I love it!

• Turn left onto Rue Croix des Petits Champs and amble over to No. 46, *Avril Gau*, creator of the Parisian's favorite minimalist bags and shoes. *So chic, ma chérie!* Well, it's nearly 1:00 P.M., my dear. I don't know about you, but for

HISTORY
By the mid-nineteenth century, Paris boasted 150 commercial galleries that cut through its palaces. Even today, visitors can take an enjoyable stroll through these charming locations known only to connoisseurs, filled with fashion boutiques and artisans' workshops, antique dealers and bistros. These glass-covered galleries are decorated with Neoclassical stucco work and have mosaic floors, an example being the Galerie Vivienne in the 2nd arrondissement, which first opened in 1826.

me shopping always works up an appetite. Let's backtrack to No. 43, *Les fines Gueules*, my favorite eatery in this neighborhood. Glad I phoned them yesterday. It's always best to reserve the day before. This place is an absolute joy for those who really like good French food: try the steak tartare of Limousine steer or the bluefin tuna tartare, both are super!

• Not too full for a couple more hours of shopping? Great! We're back to No. 10 Place des Victoires, to "le must of the must," called simply *Victoire* (what else?). This is a store we return to, season in, season out, because they make us feel so at home. The collections are gorgeous and varied: fad, classic, city casual, or dressy. They also have eccentric and must-have accessories, not to mention fun things for ephemeral occasions and designer fashions in timeless styles. Next stop is *Maje* to shop for casual wear that is simple but feminine. Just ravishing!

• Walk for about a minute or two down a little street called Rue Vide-Gousset to the Place des Petits-Pères. On the way, you'll see the Notre-Dame des Victoires basilica and, at No. 4 Place des Petits Pères, you'll discover a surprising florist called *Sylvain George*, specializing in orchids, of which he offers more than sixty types! It is so interesting when Sylvain talks about his flowers ... a real botany lesson! At No. 6 there's a shop called *Maison Bleue*, a novel concept store offering a remarkable mélange of old and new jewelry, vintage accessories, and select creations by young designers such as *Petite Mendigote*, *Les Cerises de Mars*, but also *Nat & Nin*, and *Delphine B1*. Upstairs, you'll find *Maison Bleue*'s designer hair salon.

• Follow Rue des Petits-Champs to your right until you spot the enchanting entrance to the Galerie Vivienne. Take in the Neoclassical décor. What atmosphere! At the entrance to the gallery, visit the boutique of *Jacqueline Singh*, a creator of marvelous fashion jewelry. At No. 15 visit *Nathalie Garçon* for exuberant feminine creations that please Parisian actresses. At No. 25 there's *La Marelle*, a consignment shop with great bargains on luxury articles.

At No. 34 we come to the boutique of *Alexis Mabille*, the haute-couture designer loved by everyone who's anyone. At No. 26 you'll find the creations of *Catherine André*, famous for her jacquard weaves and her jerseys and shawls in stunning colors.

• Return to Rue des Petits Champs and walk down the street to visit another historical shopping arcade called Passage Choiseul. Stroll down a magical passageway from another era. Notice the glass roof and natural lighting that make this illustrious place so charming. One of my favorite shops there is No. 11, *L'Effet Bulles*, where I buy gifts, costume jewelry, and cool decorations.

• 6:00 P.M. How time flies! Back to Galerie Vivienne for our last stop, *Legrand filles & fils*, a renowned wine merchant and traditional gourmet foods shop. Here we sip a glass of fine wine in a sublime early-twentieth-century atmosphere. Relax, you have done a good job!

Silverware

Dining in Paris is often a delicate or embarrassing experience for foreigners. The French, like all people, share certain conventions that govern good manners and define what's expected in certain situations, so an individual can be "positioned" in relation to the norm. Unlike in the United States, England, and many other countries, including Italy, where the prongs of forks and spoons face upward, when setting a table in the "French way," forks and spoons must be placed facing downward. According to a popular saying, if you place forks facing upward, it is seen as "an attack on your guests." Now that Paris has become such a cosmopolitan city, we see all types of silverware and table settings, but the Parisian woman is attached, by tradition and education, to her "French way" of setting a table even if she now applies it in its simplest form.

What silverware to use and how?

LINKS
• Luxury
• Seating
• Table

• For fish. Use the fish fork and fish knife; if you don't have a fish knife, never use the regular knife but a piece of bread instead. Try to remove all the bones before eating. If you have to take a bone out of your mouth, put it on your fork preferably, then on the edge of your plate.

• For smoked salmon. Butter a piece of toast. Squeeze a few drops of lemon juice onto the salmon on your plate then cut a piece with the fish knife. Put it in your mouth with the fork and eat the buttered bread.

• For oysters. Using the small oyster fork, detach the flesh of the oyster from the shell and bring it to your mouth. You can drink the seawater in the shell but delicately without making any noise.

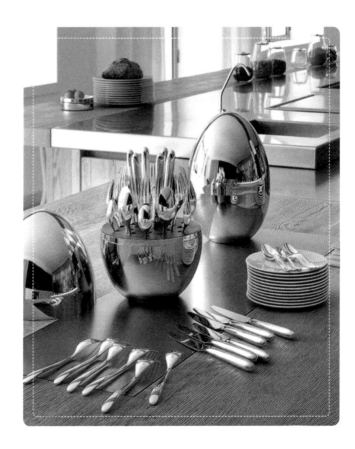

MY TIP
In Paris, you "push" bits of meat and vegetables onto the fork with a piece of bread, not with the knife.

• For salad. In Paris, you never cut salad with your knife. Fold the salad leaves with the fork and a piece of bread and then put them in your mouth. But normally, the hostess prepares the salad so that guests can eat bite-sized bits of salad and don't have to contend with forking over-sized leaves into their mouths.

• For cheese. You must never touch cheese with your fingers. Use a piece of bread to hold the cheese and remove the crust with your knife. Don't use a fork, even if you're given one!

• For asparagus. For a formal home-cooked dinner, the hostess should trim and prepare asparagus, so that it can be eaten entirely. Traditionally, asparagus should be cut with your fork and then dipped in the sauce in your plate. Among friends, you can eat it with your fingers and dip the tips in the sauce. But you are never supposed to use your knife!

• For desserts and tarts. Eat them with a fork; the spoon is used to push only the food onto the fork and to eat cream or coulis.

• For fruit. Even if it's easier, don't use your hands. Cut the fruit in half on the plate, starting from the stem, then put the flat surface face down on the plate. Keeping the fruit in place with the fork, remove the skin with the knife then remove the core and the seeds.

Sky

Like all Parisian women, I just love looking at the Paris sky! Watching its colors change with the seasons in the Jardins des Tuileries, at the *parvis* (courtyard) of Notre-Dame, or on the banks of the Seine. The Paris sky is a work of art in itself but also frames a work of art: depending on its mood, the Arènes de Lutèce, the Musée Beaubourg, the baths at Cluny, the Opéra, the Tour Eiffel, the Grand Palais, or the Champs Elysées have a different kind of luminosity. When the sky is gray, the monuments

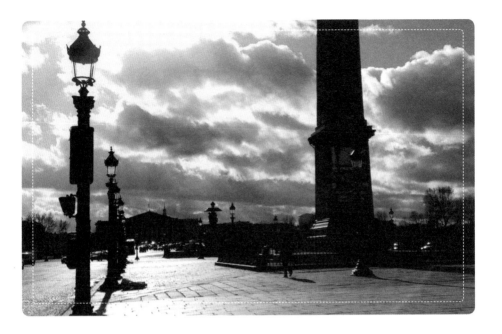

of Paris take center stage, but when the weather is good, the dense blue sky becomes the star of the urban landscape. In the winter, the low sky bathes the damp roofs in gray, with only a few stray hints of light barely brightening the mood. A storm breaks out; the sky is heavy, oppressive, and cruel. The sky is unhappy and Paris suffers. Feeling sad, the Parisian dons her little black dress. To gain forgiveness, the sky offers her a beautiful rainbow. Photographers and artists go crazy. The rest of the year, the sky is gray and white with wisps of gray, the sun hides, appears weakly then disappears, lightly tinting a few surrounding clouds with yellow. Feeling melancholy, the Parisian dresses in gray. On good days, when the sun has been shining, the Paris sky is dominated by blue and its many and varied washed-out tones, but the clouds, slightly more transparent than usual, are still there. Feeling happy, the Parisian puts on her trench coat and goes out for a walk. And then, when we're least expecting it, here comes the great big blue sky, deep, intense, and cloudless!

Incredible, it's February, June, or October and no one was expecting it. Full of excitement, the Parisian hurriedly puts on her white pants and pumps and goes onto the terrace to enjoy the irrepressible joy that this incredible blue Parisian sky brings her. "The weather's always so good in Paris," she'll tell her cousin in Bordeaux.

Les oiseaux du Bon Dieu, viennent du monde entier, pour bavarder entre eux (The good Lord's birds come from the world over to chat amongst themselves), sang Edith Piaf. There's definitely something special about our Paris sky!

Snob

"Behind her snobbish and cold appearance, the most fascinating and charming city in the world is, instead, snobbish and cold." Paradoxical, is it not? And yet it is more or less what they say about Paris "across the border." But why are Parisian women so moody, bad tempered, never happy, and stuck up? Is it perhaps "old-fashioned" to display a disenchanted and mute face? Or is it too much stress, too many demands, lack of sun or sleep, and the weight of the stereotypical *grandeur* of France? Or maybe the fact of living in Paris makes them feel superior to the rest of the world? We are fortunate to live in the "City of Lights," incredibly beautiful and culturally rich, but our character tends toward grayness and skepticism. But there is a magic trick that can change things. Those that get to know us discover that we are sophisticated people with values and true human qualities, with a highly developed sense of friendship and an incredible spirit of solidarity, which was once again demonstrated at the historic march for freedom on January 2015. So? I often tell my foreign friends who complain about Parisian snobbery not to stop at the first inhospitable and unfriendly contact but to go beyond. We love to throw ourselves into everything we undertake and we put more enthusiasm into a relationship that might last than in a

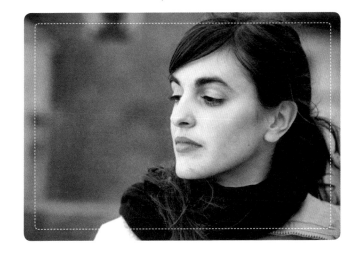

momentary contact that may have no future. That said, it is true that Paris has exaggeratedly snobbish codes of conduct. But isn't that the case in all big cities? Although perhaps a little stereotypical, this is, unfortunately, what I have noticed while watching my city. I hope that Generation Z Parisian women, born in the twenty-first century, will be more relaxed while preserving their charm and their mystery. In any case, good news for tourists: kindness and courtesy are "twee" and fashionable in Paris now and we hope that this sweet trend will take root.

How to be a snob, in general:

• Strike a distinctly bored attitude, a mix of sulking and disappointment.
• Criticize and never be satisfied.
• Never be cheerful.

How to be a snob, specifically:

• Accompany cheese with a white wine and not a traditional red (why not?).
• Have issue No. 18 of the super-elitist and erratic magazine *Égoïste* on the coffee table (No. 17 is from 2015).
• Visit the museums of Paris at night (you don't have time to see them during the day!).
• If she can't see all the exhibitions, a good Parisian

woman must at least know all the programs.
- Talk about your Little Black Dress in English or LBD (more chic than the French *Petite Robe Noire*).
- Serve sardines with a fine wine.
- Drink plenty of tea and infusions (good for your skin and figure!).
- Drink only certain brands of champagne and criticize the others.
- Wear vintage (like everywhere else).
- Love contemporary art, and always keep yourself informed about big events in Basel, Venice, Miami, and Paris, of course.
- Savor chocolate as if it were fine wine and talk about it.
- Use a lot of English words—"so chic," "glam," "IT-girl"— and typical Parisian expressions.
- Decline an invitation to a party because you've been invited to two others for the same evening.
- Say "no" to meat and eat only ethical and fair-trade food.
- Follow the Mediterranean diet.
- Put ice cubes in champagne (see the entry "Champagne" for what I think about ...).

Suitcase

We're talking about the bag the Parisian packs when she travels and the bag you should pack when you come to Paris ... Aside from her basics, the Parisian woman puts a lot of thought into packing her bag to make absolutely sure she doesn't forget anything or take things she doesn't need, which can spoil the vacation. With a few exceptions, she often starts figuring out what to take at least three days before leaving. There are fans of to-take lists, lovers of monochrome "white in the summer, black the rest of the time" paired with versatile accessories, and minimalists— "I take the absolute minimum, the basics." For women travelers the world over, packing a bag is a real ordeal— you never know exactly what to take, what the weather

will be like, you're always afraid of forgetting something important and having to make concessions. That said, the Parisian tries to observe a few basic rules she was taught by her mother and grandmother:
• Always dress up rather than down.
• Plain rather than patterned.
• Never travel with valuables.
• Take garments that don't crease too much.
• Bring a versatile little cardigan for evening dresses.
• No duplicates (she really wants to take her latest *Equipment* blouse or her new *Vanessa Bruno* dress, but it's decision time—we expect, however, that's not the last we'll see of her favorite new clothes).

On your visit to Paris, you'll be captivated by the *Ville Lumière*, but don't count on bright sunshine! Better to be surprised, which happens more often than you might

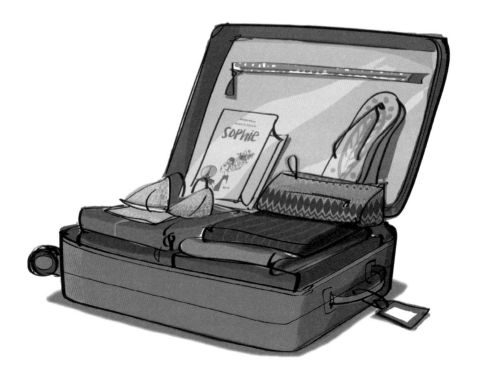

think (about 160 days a year). Think practical but stylish clothes you can go out in and feel good in despite the rain or cold. The ideal is to think about layering, which is trendy in Paris. This means you can add or take things off depending on the temperature and the whims of the sky— hence the idea of monochrome or varying tones of one color. The risk of a heat wave in Paris is minimal, so limit light garments in favor of practical ones (keep in mind that you'll be walking up to five miles a day to make the most of all the wonderful things the city has to offer). As for elegance, no need to bring ten evening dresses. To look chic in Paris, go for simplicity and sophistication. The always-glamorous little black dress will be perfect, just accessorize it differently every evening. Plus shopping in Paris is an art that's great fun to practice. So as not to overload your bag, wear your bulky sneakers (stylish or black) and outerwear, even if you have to layer. And, most importantly, limit the size of your bag; apartments in Paris are small and lack storage! One of the best techniques for saving space in your bag is to fold then roll your clothes and use belts, socks or leggings, and underwear to fill the gaps. If you're coming to Paris for only three or four days, just bring a carry-on bag so you avoid the interminable wait at the airport, and always bring some extra underwear in case your luggage is lost!

Sun

In the *Ville Lumière* as elsewhere, the absence of sunshine is synonymous with gloom and periods of depression. It's really true: the barometer of our mood varies according to the whims of the sun. The proof is that, in Paris, where the gray is omnipresent, a sunny day is always a beautiful day! We Parisian women are so hungry for light and sun that the sunlight gives us joy. It is a need that also has a scientific basis: the sun on the skin stimulates the molecules of pleasure and well-being and is also essential

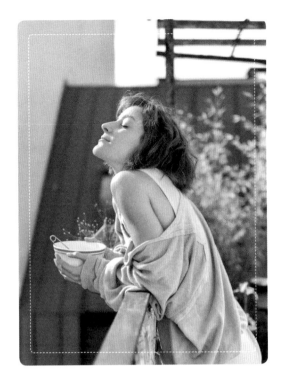

for the synthesis of vitamin D. Haven't you seen Parisian women sitting at a sidewalk café with their chins lifted toward the sky to catch some sunshine?

Sunset

One of the Parisian woman's favorite things to do, and possibly the most romantic, is to watch the sun set, as the last shafts of daylight illuminate the Paris rooftops, the sky turns crimson, and the Tour Eiffel, the bridges, the trees, the dome of the Grand Palais, and the *Horses of Marly* gradually become silhouetted against a multicolored backdrop. Where's the best spot to watch this spectacle? It's not easy to be at the right place at this time; we're often stuck in a traffic jam, at work, or waiting at the

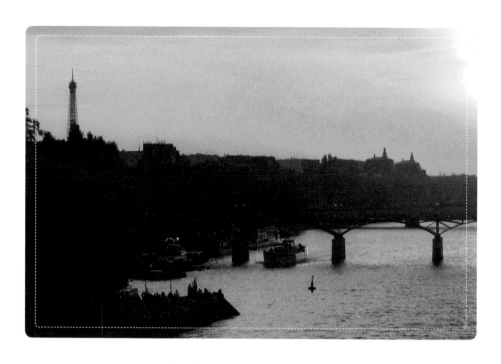

MY TIP
There's nothing like
a twilight cruise on the
Seine. You can admire
the monuments set
against a multicolored
sky and then the lights
of Paris as night falls.
This is what we did
for our wedding
reception; my family
and friends were moved
and enthralled by the
beauty of the *Ville
Lumière* seen from
the river.

school gates. Amandine lives near the Tour Montparnasse.
Its 689-foot-high terrace is a fantastic place to admire
the sun setting behind the Tour Eiffel, with a panoramic
view over the entire capital. Clémence, who works in the
Opéra district, climbs to the top floor of the Printemps
Haussmann department store to admire the spectacular
twilight views over Montmartre, the Grand Palais, the Tour
Eiffel, the Arc de Triomphe, and the Défense. Lisa has her
painting studio on Montmartre hill. She regularly goes
to sit with her sweetheart on the steps of the Parvis
du Sacré Coeur, the high point of the city, to watch
the Paris sky turning crimson—it's an ultra-romantic
atmosphere with street music, enthralled tourists, and
a panoramic view of Paris. I work on the Right Bank and
live on the Left. When the sun's setting, I'm riding my bike
across one of the bridges of Paris—the Pont Neuf or Pont
Alexandre III. From there, it's a majestic spectacle, as the
Seine takes on a bright orange-red glow and the last rays
of sunshine light up the monuments. On the weekend,

I take my children, Marcel and Emma, to the Passerelle des Arts to view this extraordinary spectacle, stretching from the Tour Eiffel and the Grand Palais on one side to the Île de la Cité on the other. Wow! And then there are the classics: taking a photo of the Tour Eiffel from the Trocadéro gardens or, the opposite, taking in the 360-degree panoramic view of Paris from the top of the Tour Eiffel. If you're lucky enough to have an apartment or a hotel room with a panoramic terrace, the best thing of all is, of course, to admire the sun setting over Paris in good company with a little glass of champagne! So Parisian.

Supermarket

Shopping right can be hard, especially if you have a big family to feed and not much time. Sometimes your neighborhood supermarket is more convenient, because you're in a rush or need bulky household products. But when she can, the *Parisienne* buys as little as possible at the big retailers.

Today's Parisian woman is well aware of the dangers of overusing industrial products, which can be hazardous to her health. This is reflected in so many popular publications by nutritionists and other scientific writers, advising us to make the right choices when we shop for food.

Buying wholesome products, and knowing where they come from, is not just fashionable, it's become a priority for our health and well-being. "When we can, we stay away from the supermarket other than for a few brand name foods we're hooked on, like *Lindt* chocolate or *Calin* low-cal yogurt. For the rest of our groceries, we try and go to our cheese shop, our baker, our greengrocer, and so forth. We go to specialists we trust, who don't use artificial colors or preservatives."

Nadège, Rue de Buci, January 16

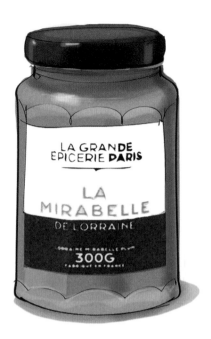

The temples of taste … The Parisian woman loves specialty grocery stores where the products are tastefully presented and selected for their quality. They are also places to visit on the weekend for those who want to meet as many friends as possible and chat! *La Grande Épicerie de Paris,* the culinary annex of *Le Bon Marché Rive Gauche*, is the cool supermarket in the 6th and 7th arrondissements. Recently, a new store opened for business in the 16th arrondissement, on Rue de Passy. Great news! It resembles an "all-in-one" market where she can find hard-to-find products from around the world, plus the service and valuable, useful advice of her trusted cheese seller and wine seller. Here we buy our *bottarga*, our *Calasparra* rice, our Italian *Rostello* ham, and our Swedish *Ramlösa* mineral water. The Parisian has reduced her consumption of meat, but when she buys it she wants quality, and the butcher shop and delicatessen/rôtisserie in *La Grande Épicerie* are the best! *Lafayette Gourmet* is THE luxury supermarket, with an adjoining tasting space, frequented by gourmets of the Rive Droite. Here the Parisian buys quality fruit and vegetables, deli meats, and the cereals and seeds that are so fashionable.

T

Table

In Paris meals remain an institution and "taking one's place at the table" is a habit that has now become an integral part of the education of even the youngest children. It allows mothers to pass on to their children the art of dining etiquette as well as healthy eating habits. Meals may well be faster than they used to be, but rituals continue to be respected. Culinary transformations, changing lifestyles, technical innovations in terms of how

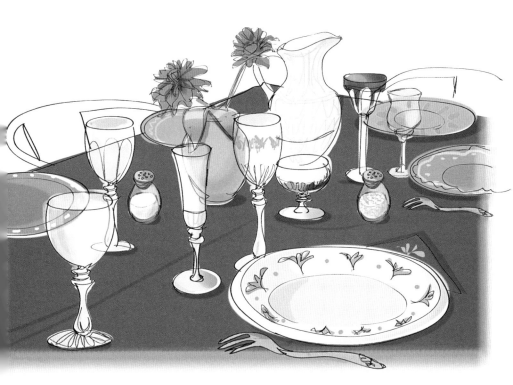

we consume food—table service has evolved in Paris as
it has in the rest of the world. Although the importance
of the dining room may have waned somewhat, it's
inversely proportional to the increasing importance
of the kitchen as a living environment. Indeed, grand
"French-style" service is gradually evolving. Tradition
is nevertheless being preserved in terms of behavior,
especially when it comes to serving and eating. Have
you ever found yourself in front of a plate of foie gras or
asparagus, asking yourself: "Now what do I do?" Under
"Silverware" and "Foie Gras" I explain the *so very French*
way of eating these complicated dishes.

Table Seating

The problem that every hostess faces: how not to slight
anyone and please everyone with the right arrangement
at the table? In Paris, like anywhere else, a sit-down dinner
doesn't inevitably require a protocol. It's not like a Parisian
woman has her boss or an elder of the church for dinner
every day, let alone the President of the Republic.
She's normally hosting her dear friends. Her greatest
concern to ensure success when organizing a dinner
is to arrange guests at the table according to their
affinities—their tastes, interests, opinions, or personalities.
If, however, she has to think about a more serious seating
arrangement for a "formal" dinner at home, at an elegant
restaurant, or at a wedding, a gala, or a charity event,
the Parisian woman will follow some basic rules of good
manners. First of all, she will organize her guest list
in a declining hierarchy based on social position and age.
In the "French" seating arrangement, the hosts sit facing
each other at the center of the table (since the ends
of the table are the most undesirable seats, they can
ALSO sit there themselves to avoid making other diners
take them). Then she will put the first man on the list
to her right, the second to her left, and will do the same

thing with the women on the list and the man of the house (opposite her). If unmarried, the hostess must never face a married man—only a parent or a girlfriend.

The clergy are the only exception: they take precedence over all the other guests and preside at the table together with the hostess. The other diners are seated according to their rank and responsibilities. Avoid seating members of the same family next to one another. Preparation, grace, and naturalness are the ABC's of every Parisian hostess in Paris, and that is why she always determines the seating arrangement before her guests arrive. She can tell each guest where to sit with apparent spontaneity and avoid gaffes. Did you know that, in order to give her guests the option of refusing the invitation, she has to tell them the names of everyone else invited?

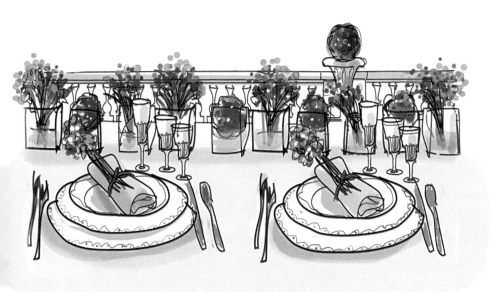

Terrace

In Paris, what we call a "terrace" can be two slightly different things:
• An open space that extends a home (but also a hotel room, etc.) toward the outside. It would be the equivalent of the terrace of a penthouse, the "rooftop."
• A kind of veranda completely open or closed by a glass wall; the outside of a bistro, café, or restaurant that opens directly onto the street. There is the Parisian concept of sitting *en terrasse*, to see and be seen or just be outdoors! The climate certainly does not predispose Paris to be one of the capitals of this type of *terrasse*, or open-air venue. Although many cities worldwide, particularly in Italy, boast a lot more, Parisian sidewalk tables have a character all their own. Elsewhere they are considered

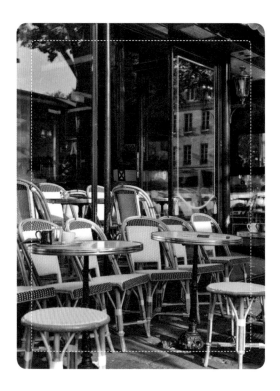

mere meeting places, while in Paris they are real open-
air theaters. The Parisian woman sits in the front row
to watch the world go by—confused tourists, embracing
lovers, moms rushing to pick up their children from
school, nervous people waiting for someone running
late, a hurried woman fighting with a heel stuck between
cobblestones, a VIP or a star who passes while chatting
with a friend. Sidewalk tables are the ideal place to study
this strange mixture of Parisians up close, a quick waltz
in which dancers of all kinds enter and leave the scene.
Remember, though, that if you can see everyone from a
sidewalk table, they can also see you! There is, however,
no need for opera glasses—everything is under control! So
when you sit at the table of a *terrasse*, it's not like sitting at
the bar, hidden under large sunglasses, for a quick coffee.
Parisians have a spirit of observation enhanced by a very
developed critical sense that is attentive to your look, who
you associate with, and what you say—if you are gossiping,
nearby ears are always alert. The sidewalk table is a salon.
Each quarter has its own, and the trick is picking one that
offers an interesting or spectacular program: a good mix
of genres, with non-stop traffic on the street or in the café.
I must say that I never tire of the outdoor tables at *Chez
Francis* in Place de l'Alma. Its strategic location between
Avenue Montaigne and Avenue George V, in front of the
Tour Eiffel and the Seine, makes it a first-rate seat for
watching pedestrians, fashion victims, businessmen—in
short, a nice mix. Timeless are the sidewalk tables of the
famous cafés in Saint-Germain-des-Prés, especially if you
like "star watching," seeing VIPs, and being seen! It's not
bad watching the patrons of *Café Madeleine*—women who
shop at the big department stores meet those who work or
live in the quarter and the tourists passing through—and
those of *Café Beaubourg*, a great place to watch visitors
to the *Centre Georges Pompidou*!
Paris is not New York and rooftop terraces are rare. Each
year, with the arrival of summer, the city unveils new
ones with stunning views of Paris. If you don't already

know them, make note of some of these magical places: *Wanderlust* on the Quai d'Austerlitz, *Quarante Trois Cocktail Bar* on the roof of the *Notre-Dame Holiday Inn,* the outdoor bar of *Peninsula* on Avenue Kleber, *Les Ombres* above the Branly museum, and, one of my favorites, the beautiful terrace of *Raphael*, a roof garden with a panoramic view of Paris and the Tour Eiffel.

The Best

LINKS
• Baguette
• Cheese
• Chocolate
• The Place to Be

The Parisian woman loves the idea of buying "nothing but the best." That goes for edibles like macaroons and baguettes and just about everything else: borders and trims, lampshades, upholstery fabrics, and silverware. The approach may come off as a little bit "stuck up," but it's legitimate if it's really based on the concept of quality. The *Parisienne* can be heard saying things like: "I eat only *Isigny* butter, and I buy cheese only at *Barthélémy's*, on Rue de Grenelle."

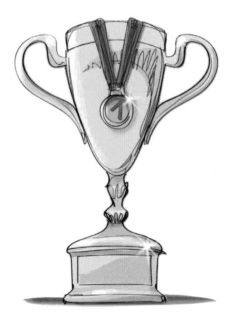

HISTORY

* The annual *Meilleurs Ouvriers de France* (Best Artisans in France) competition was founded in 1924 to recognize the best craftsmen in a number of specialties. Three *Meilleurs Ouvriers de France* 2015 to discover in Paris: Virginie Basselot, chef at the *Saint-James Hotel* (the second woman to win this coveted award since the competition's founding in 1924); *Kevin Chambenoit,* Restaurant Director at the *Bristol Hotel* (*Meilleur Ouvrier de France* in the *Maître d'Hôtel* category); and *Jérôme Chaucesse,* Master Pastry Chef at the *Crillon Hotel* who has reigned over the dessert menu there since 2004 (his cakes are exquisite poetry).

"I buy my chocolate macaroons only at *Ladurée,* the best macaroon baker of the Rive Gauche."

"Charcuterie? Only at *Gilles Vérot,* medal of honor in 1998 for his *andouille de Vire,* first prize of honor that year for his *andouillette de Troyes.*"

"I buy my bread in the 15th arrondissement at *Frédéric Lalos*'s bakery. He is a *Meilleur Ouvrier de France,** and his baguette is simply incredible."

"The best Bellini cocktail in Paris," someone told me last night at a reception, "is made by *Colin Peter Field,* the head bartender at the Ritz."

The Place to Be

Namely: "Being in the right place at the right time." Whether in Paris or elsewhere, the Parisian woman is keen on always being in the right place at the right time! Restaurants, bars, cultural or social events—she is aware of everything that is happening in her city and organizes her forays with *savoir-faire.* The "right place" often has a connotation more exclusive than trendy, places known by a select few, for "real gourmets" or "connoisseurs." And she is one, of course.

So, trendy restaurants are not necessarily her favorite places. Although she doesn't disdain occasionally attending the great, always fashionable classics—*Hôtel Costes, Ralph's, Avenue,* or the terrace of *L'Esplanade*—let's be clear, she will never, ever go to dinner at a restaurant that is too "has been." Out! On the other hand, she is eclectic, she likes (or would like!) to go to *Arpège*, the restaurant of *Alain Passard*, which she considers one of the best French restaurants (a definition that normally horrifies the rest of France), but loves excellent bistros. And then she has her regulars: *La Cigale Récamier* in the 6th arrondissement; *Chez Fernand* on Rue Guisarde for the *boeuf Bourguignon;* and *Closerie de Lilas*, where she feels good enough to have lunch alone! In fact, the Parisian woman's address book is full of confidential and personal niches, all very decent and current. One of my favorites: *Hôtel*, in the 6th arrondissement—a cozy salon once frequented by Oscar Wilde and Serge Gainsbourg. With my girlfriends, I like to go to *Fontaine de Mars* or, on Saturdays, to *La Cantine de Merci*, on Boulevard Beaumarchais.

The latest trend of the moment: luxury bars—from high-design ones to those richly decorated with period wainscoting. Parisian women love to have a drink before going to dinner. With her husband, a girlfriend for a chat, for a pick-me-up, or to criticize the last opening, or with a "possible future" boyfriend ... Whether it's *Glass*, the new bar now fashionable in the So-Pi (South Pigalle) quarter, *Café Marly* to sip a cocktail at sunset in front of the Pyramide du Louvre or the "très, très chic" *Bar 8* of *Mandarin Oriental*, there's no lack of places. To be worthy of a Parisian woman, it should be "in but exclusive." *Costes* is ok, but it is "too popular with jet setters and tourists." For my part, I love the *Patio Bar* of the *Prince de Galles*! Whether she is passionate about contemporary art (a *must* in Paris) or sports, the Parisian woman's date book will follow that of the big events. *FIAC* (International Fair of Contemporary Art) or *Roland Garros* is a mandatory trip— but on the right day. Real chic consists of knowing *where* to go and *when*. It's very difficult to know, because the "in" and "out" list is constantly changing. One thing is certain: we can't miss some of the big shows, and it is essential to go on opening day, especially when it comes to the

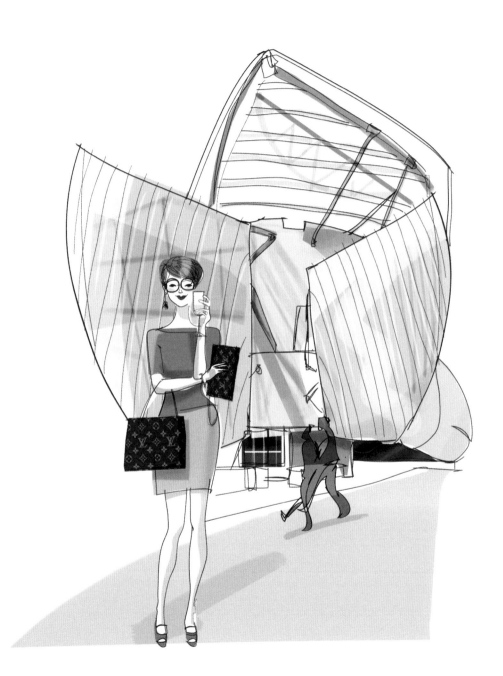

Fondation Louis Vuitton or *Musée d'Art Moderne de la Ville de Paris*. Paris is an innovative, bold, and vibrant city, where something is always happening. From *Fashion Week* to *Dîner en Blanc* or the *Prix de Diane*, the *Vendanges Montaigne*, the premiere of the Opéra Bastille, or the opening of *Paris Photo*, there's no lack of social events. Telling you where to go and when is difficult because the *right place* changes too quickly. Following the Parisian woman's migration in the heart of her city requires arming yourself with patience and finding a good local expert informed on current events.

The Tie

The Parisian woman loves well-dressed men and loves buying ties for her guy, lots and lots of them. She's a real master at this and very rarely makes the wrong choice. Her secret? Whether she's lazy, practical, in love, or in too much of a rush, her technique is infallible: she opens the closet and looks at what he has:
"Nothing but blue."
"He must like blue."
"I'm going to buy a blue tie and if he doesn't like it, he can change it."
There's no point in choosing a tie that matches your dress or the color of his eyes or, worse, purple, because it's in vogue. Your man, like 90% of the male sex, sticks to a particular style. If he likes blue ties, he's not likely to wear an orange one to make you happy; he'll wear only blue of varying shades with different designs, but always a variation on blue. If he wears only narrow gray ties, it's because he likes them; it's a waste of time forcing him to change! And, hello! This is what Parisian women have known for a very long time. So, follow the example and nothing will prevent you from borrowing the tie in question for yourself, to flaunt a Marlene Dietrich-type sexy look!

MY TIP

"The tie must stand out against the suit and the shirt without clashing," recommends my friend Maurizio Marinella, the "king" of the Italian tie and president of *E. Marinella*. "It must be of a color darker than the shirt and more intense than the jacket. It's often the only colored note of serious clothing, but pay attention not to exaggerate! Always avoid having a too studied and affected comprehensive look and opt for a *decontractée* (relaxed) elegance. Never a coordinated tie and small pocket handkerchief: it is as useless as anachronistic affectation." *Ipse dixit!*

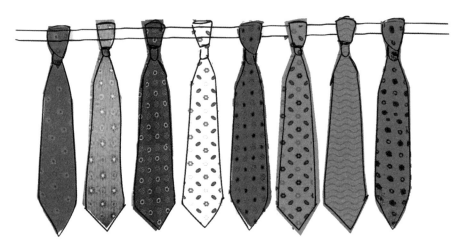

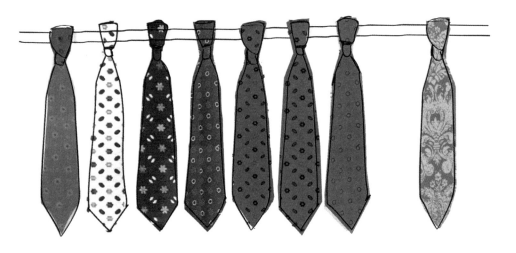

THE RECIPE

Even certain recipes are vintage. They go back to food traditions that are somewhat snubbed today, because they're not exactly what you'd call ... dietetic! But the Parisian woman likes to amaze her guests, and every now and then she makes this truly mouthwatering dish.

Onion soup gratinéed with cheese

Serves 4
5 large onions sliced
6 tbsp. butter
1 tbsp. flour
6 cups stock or water
1/3 cup grated Gruyère cheese
toasted bread
salt, pepper

In a pressure cooker brown the thinly sliced onions in 2 1/4 tablespoons of butter. Sprinkle with a heaping tablespoon of flour, stirring with a wooden spoon until the roux is slightly brown. Gradually add 6 cups of water or cold stock and continue to stir, making sure the mixture doesn't stick to the bottom, until it boils. Salt and pepper. Seal the cooker with its lid and bring it to pressure over high heat. As soon as the valve whistles reduce the heat and cook for 15 minutes. Brown the slices of bread in a skillet with the leftover butter, then place in a soup tureen that's oven safe. Pour the soup over the toasted bread. Top with grated Gruyère. Gratinée a few seconds in individual bowls or in a baking dish.

she passionately cultivates the traditions of the past, something that, as always, gives her a certain vintage "arty-trad" style. To express herself as a unique being, she no longer buys predictable or mass-produced objects. That's too trivial and boring. She loves exclusivity and an object that stands out from the others, and vintage addresses this need. Something that's in with both women and modern men.

Walk in Paris

Timeless and contemporary, artistic and cultural, glamorous and romantic ... Paris has enormous appeal and seductive power for both tourists and Parisian women who constantly use it as the backdrop for the filming of their love life: walks along the banks of the Seine,

intimate moments under the chestnut trees on the Place Dauphine, nighttime meetings on the *parvis* of Notre-Dame, interminable kisses on public benches, strolling hand-in-hand through gardens, or proposals in unusual places. Paris never ceases to amaze her and inspire her dreams. With its little streets, secret passages, and charming squares, it's THE romantic city par excellence, the ideal setting for the eternal romantic in the Parisian woman. Here are a few of our favorite adventures:
• Strolling through the bohemian side streets of Montmartre, climbing up the steps of the butte

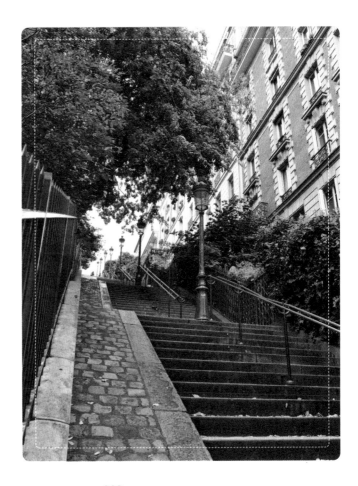

MY TIP

When it's really cold, you can take shelter in the big hothouses of the Jardin des Plantes, far from the hum of the city—simply magnificent! For a wonderful memory, in black and white, go to the Place de l'Hôtel de Ville to reproduce the mythical lovers' kiss photographed in 1950 by Robert Doisneau.

If attaching "a love padlock" to the railings of the Pont des Arts was so far the goal of a romantic walk, this is no longer possible, because the weight of all those padlocks has jeopardized the bridge security.

to the Sacré-Coeur Basilica then having a little ride on the carousel in the pretty Place des Abbesses, where time seems to have stood still.

• Walking through the narrow streets of Le Marais to see the city's oldest monuments, including Victor Hugo's house on the Place des Vosges, and get a sense of the romanticism of the seventeenth century.

• Doing some shopping with your sweetheart, hand in hand, in the picturesque Mouffetard district, known as "la Mouffe," which looks just like a village of the past with its old houses and maze of little streets.

• Declaring your love right at the tip of the Square du Vert-Galant on the Île de la Cité, one of the most beautiful places in the city, or organizing picnics or drinks with friends there in the summer.

• Strolling under the bridges to the Pont Marie, nicknamed the "lovers' bridge," to make a wish (the arches symbolize union, and only the water of the river hears the cooing of the doves), or through the Jardin de Fontenay des Archives Nationales to share confidences away from listening ears in a romantic nineteenth-century setting.

• Whispering sweet nothings on the banks of Canal Saint-Martin, with its romantic bridges and footbridges and its magical atmosphere, taking you away from your everyday routine.

• Kissing on a public bench in the Jardin des Tuileries, the favored place for dalliances—in times past, its path and walks were the theater in which games of love and chance were played—or by the Medici fountain in the Jardin du Luxembourg or the Arènes de Lutèce.

• Strolling along covered passageways, like the Colbert or Vivienne galleries and the Verdeau or Jouffroy passageways, enjoying the special almost "retro" atmosphere created by the glass roofs and delightful stores.

Wardrobe

I suppose that when I speak about "the" Parisian woman, I could be accused of over generalizing. I can already imagine some of my Parisian friends and neighbors reading my words and claiming that they are exceptions to the rule. But between you and me, if they say that, it is more to protect their "secret garden" and to preserve the mystery of our "spontaneous" and "natural" elegance. When I listen to my girlfriends and read what the media say about Parisian tastes, I discover with dismay that my style is not unique, that in fact I share it with a great many other women in the capital. So how does a *Parisienne* develop a distinctive personal style? One answer is *accessorization.* Another is the importance she gives to each article in her wardrobe according to her lifestyle, her personality, and her mood. Considering, with all due modesty, the compliments I've received since the age of eighteen on my look and impeccable taste, I, Sophie the Parisian, have a duty to share the do's and don'ts of putting together a wardrobe worthy of praise. The Parisian woman of taste must be elegant but not boringly classic, chic yet casual.

I like some luxury brands for their quality (not for a bling-bling monogram). This is just for the clothes I call my basics, for which I'm willing to make a long-term investment. But I also know how to shop wisely for less expensive brands, and nothing pleases me more than unearthing a bargain somewhere in the world. The principle: develop a wardrobe of quality with a mix of costly and bargain articles.

LINKS
• Avenue Montaigne
• Jeans
• Little Black Dress

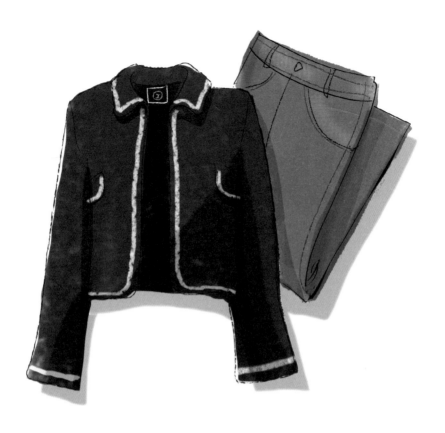

Like all Parisian women, my wardrobe and I are a love story. Expect me to throw a fit if I've mislaid my favorite white T-shirt or stained my vintage blouse. Crazy? No more so then my menfolk: witness my son's expletives when he can't find his rugby shorts or my husband's invectives when his favorite shirt is in the ironing basket (even if he has a dozen others hanging in his closet). My attitude each morning, standing before my closet, is so hypocritical and so Parisian. My first thought is conscious: "I've nothing to wear!" But I slip on whatever I've got since I'm in rush. My second thought (unconscious): "I've got to create a style. What accessories do I need to personalize my look?" My third thought is conscious. "I look too stuffy. How can I be cooler and

MY TIP
My favorite brands?
Designer names for my
"basics," big
international and
French *prêt-à-porter*
brands for seasonal
wear, and products
from retail chain stores
for my accessories.
When traveling in the
States, I love going
to *Target!*

foxier?" Undo a couple of buttons? Maybe a slightly visible push-up bra? How about a top that bares one shoulder? Finally, I artfully muss my hair to look more natural.

The words we love to hear when we take out a skirt we haven't worn for fifteen years: "Is that something new?" The words that are hazardous for our health: "The absolute must this season is …" spotted in a fashion mag.

In practice, my wardrobe is a well-balanced mix of:

• Designer clothes, big name ready-to-wear brands, and stuff from retail chain stores. Not to mention fashions picked up on sale in Italy or the south of France as well as trendy or ethnic handicrafts that add a little *je ne sais quoi* to an outfit (as long as you don't overdo it) and vintage or secondhand odds and ends.

• Timeless basics and seasonal wear. Both are purchased at advertised or private sales or from an e-tailer, but I've fallen in love with and bought things on a whim that I stumbled upon at yard sales or found at open-air markets. On rare occasions I spoil myself at a designer boutique. For we *Parisiennes*, building a wardrobe is a never-ending labor of love!

• Classics spiced up with a little extra touch, something exotic or borderline like leather pants or an animal print top that originally weren't intended for the wardrobe of a prim and proper young lady; Parisians have a talent for working unconventional articles into conventional looks. This look might be called "daring but with a safety net."

• 90% solid colors + 5% stripes + 2% flower prints + 1% polka dots + 2% other. Black, navy, ecru, gray, white, and beige. A hint of seasonal color, and of course a little blue to match my eyes (for others it will be olive green or nut brown)—a childhood habit. In fact, the "color" that really leaps out at you when you open my closet is basic black!

• Mostly pants that flatter my figure, skirts, dresses, tops in every color, lots of lingerie, lots of scarves, tailored jackets, and tons of shoes. And my jeans (in fact, I have plenty of jeans but only one pair I call MY jeans).

Wine

Living in a country of vineyards, the Parisian woman has always been accustomed to understand and speak the language of wine. Each family has its own preferences, its favorite wines, and, despite arguments between supporters of the various regions (Burgundy versus Bordeaux), the French woman in general—and the Parisian, in particular—is proud of France's wine production. She loves to talk about wine, taste it, and serve it to friends.

The French way of serving wine is an art that, like any discipline, has its rules and is more than pouring liquid into a glass. A simple ceremony but one that requires discretion and *savoir faire*, especially in Paris. One of the most common mistakes is to pour too much wine in the

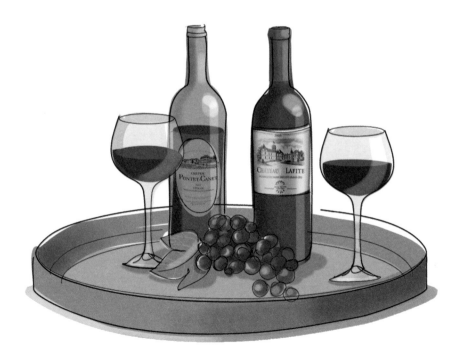

MY TIP
To appreciate wine, learn to drink it slowly, focusing a few seconds on each stage of the tasting: appearance, aroma, taste, and so on. The hostess will appreciate your curiosity and your sense of the "product," especially if it is a great wine to which you have shown sensitivity. You don't need to be a specialist; just observe and analyze what you drink based on your impressions. Like looking at a work of art, in the end your emotions are the only things that matter.

glass. One-third is more than enough—even one-quarter! Remember that wine is a drink to be enjoyed, so you want your guests to appreciate it but not get drunk! Some white wines or, in particular, champagne, are served chilled and not warm poured ten minutes before consuming.

It is important to serve the wine just before the dish and not the opposite, so that guests can appreciate the combination. Bring the wine to the table before the dish, so as to synchronize the service.

The capacity of a glass depends on the time it takes to eat the accompanying dish, since an appetizer is eaten faster than a main course. The various sizes of glasses are based on this principle. The first wine that accompanies the appetizers, whether white or red, will be served in the smallest wine glass, while the second wine, which accompanies the main dish, will be bigger, and, obviously, the biggest glass of all is for water. If the glasses are the same size, the first wine will be served in the nearest glass.

Your guests are not obliged to like or drink all the wine you have served them; it all depends on each one's personal taste and way of enjoying wine. Some people (and their number is increasing) like to taste without drinking too much, while others have no problem drinking everything that is served to them. Don't make an issue of it and just offer the next wine.

Z

Z (Generation)

Amandine, Ambre, Camille, Coline, Emma, Flora, Jade, Justine, Léa, Lisa, Manon, Marie, Nina, Sarah, Violette … The generation Z Parisian, who's about thirteen to eighteen, is a very different young woman from the stereotypical image of her elders. The crisis people start talking about when they're "young," more than being an obstacle for their future, means parents who are always complaining, and less money for vacations, clothes, and other things.

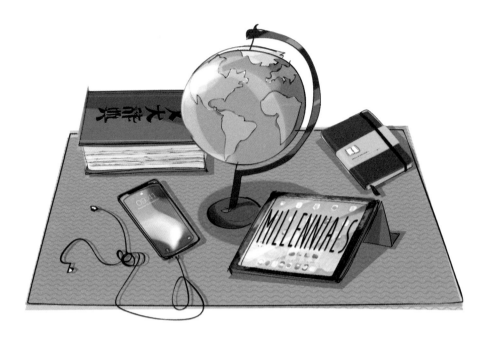

Born in this "gloomy" climate at the close of the century,
she's become hardened, and since she isn't banking
on getting any help, she'll probably have more of a chance
of doing well when she leaves school.
Smartphones, iPads and social networks have always
existed for her; the Internet helped her entertain herself
while giving her unlimited and constant access to
knowledge and sharing—a fundamental feature of her
culture. We don't know enough about her yet to guess
what she'll be doing in twenty years, but judging
from her attitude and her reactions to questions, we can
speculate: she'll be an entrepreneur, make decisions, act
quickly, and, most of all, ultra-connected, she'll be more
sociable, less individualistic, and most certainly rely
on support from the community to get on in her life.
Already, the sharing economy is her theme; collective
success motivates her and she couldn't care less about
hierarchy. The image of the chic and slim Parisian woman
interests her as much as it did earlier generations, first
and foremost on social networks, where having the right

look and the right pose are vital to exist and be accepted. Her state of mind is incredibly "open source," and her plans weren't made in the sandbox but arose from present opportunities. She's learned to forge her own opinion and gain the capacity of the self-taught. Pragmatic, she aims to become a skilled adult and wants to put her plans into practice as quickly as possible—online of course!

Whatever trials she's going to face, she declares she's ready to face the working world with a more phlegmatic approach than her big sister, who's still waiting for a job she was promised and that never comes. From what she says, her parents are only there for her equilibrium and not to map out her route for her. Her favorite expression—"Don't worry, I'll manage"—also clearly reflects her state of mind. She's not talking about her pocket money or her phone package; she just wants to make her mum understand she doesn't need to interfere in her stuff! At school, she rubs shoulders with all sorts of cultures and understands that the world is a big place but within her reach, so during the summer, when her parents' resources allow, she goes to work in Washington, Shanghai, or Sydney, but also India or South America. Although she's confident about the future, she knows she's got a part to play in getting what she wants to become reality and doesn't want to wait until she's forty to realize her dreams. But it must not be at any price. For her, success means "being happy at work and at home."

Being a Parisian woman today means being aware that the Parisian woman of the future will be a long way away from the clichés and image we have of her today. Thanks for taking the time to read!

See you soon,
Sophie

Paris, October 1, 2018

Sophie's Addresses

DELI SHOPS

Bakeries
Paul
77 Rue de Seine
75006 | +33 1 55 42 02 23

Boulangerie Dupain
20 Boulevard des
Filles du Calvaire
75011 | +33 1 58 30 72 36

Gontran Cherrier
22 Rue Caulaincourt
75018 | +33 1 46 06 82 66

Cheese
Laurent Dubois Maubert
47ter Boulevard
Saint-Germain
75005 | +33 1 43 54 50 93

Michel Sanders
4 Rue Lobineau
75006 | +33 1 46 34 05 94
Barthélemy
51 Rue de Grenelle
75007 | +33 1 42 22 82 24

Marie-Anne Cantin
12, Rue du
Champ-de-Mars
75007 | +33 1 45 50 43 94

Chez Virginie
54 Rue Damrémont
75018 |+33 1 46 06 76 54

Chocolate
Jacques Genin
133 Rue de Turenne
75003 |+33 1 45 77 29 01

Cyril Lignac
34 Rue du Dragon
75006 | +33 1 55 87 21 40

Patrick Roger
3 Place de la Madeleine
75008 | +33 9 67 08 24 47

Pastry Shops
Sitron
15 Rue Marie Stuart
75002 | +33 1 40 20 92 31

Les Fées Pâtissières
21 Rue Rambuteau
75004 | +33 1 42 77 42 15

Arnaud Larher
93 Rue de Seine
75006 | + 33 1 43 29 38 15

Gérard Mulot
76 Rue de Seine
75006 | +33 1 43 26 85 77

Ladurée
21 Rue Bonaparte
75006 | +33 1 44 07 64 87

La Maison du Chou
7 Rue de Furstenberg
75006 | +33 9 54 75 06 05

Les Bonbons
6 Rue de Bréa
75006 | +33 1 43 26 21 15

L'éclair de Génie
13 Rue de
l'Ancienne Comédie
75006 | +33 1 84 79 23 44

Pierre Hermé
72 Rue Bonaparte
75006 | +33 1 43 54 47 77

Des gâteaux et du pain
89 Rue du Bac
75007 | +33 6 98 95 33 18

Gâteaux Thoumieux
58 Rue St-Dominique
75007 | +33 1 45 51 12 12

FASHION AND BEAUTY

Jovoy Parfums Rares
4 Rue de Castiglione
75001 | +33 1 40 20 06 19

Kabuki
23-25 Rue Étienne Marcel
75001 | +33 1 42 33 55 65

Alexis Mabille
34 Galerie Vivienne
75002 | +33 9 80 62 92 70

Maison Bleue
5 Place des Petits-Pères
75002 | +33 1 44 50 54 80

Nathalie Garçon
15-17 Galerie Vivienne
75002 | +33 1 40 20 14 00

Nose
20 Rue Bachaumont
75002 | +33 1 40 26 46 03

Repetto
22, Rue de la Paix
75002 | +33 1 44 71 83 12

Victoire
10 Place des Victoires
75002 | +33 1 49 27 94 76

Azzedine Alaïa Stock
18 Rue de la Verrerie
75004 | +33 1 42 72 19 19

La Piscine
13 Rue des
Francs-Bourgeois
75004 | +33 1 48 87 59 24

Aigle
139 Boulevard
Saint-Germain
75006 |+33 1 46 33 26 23

Emmanuelle Zysman
33 Rue de Grenelle
75007 | +33 1 42 22 05 57

Montaigne Market
33 Rue François 1er
75008 | +33 1 53 67 64 75

APC Surplus
20 Rue André Del Sarte
75018 | +33 1 42 62 10 88

Spree
16 Rue La Vieuville
75018 | +33 1 42 23 41 40

Nous
48 Rue Cambon
75001 | +33 1 40 28 40 75

HOME

Flowers
Maison Vertumne
12 Rue de la Sourdière
75001 | +33 1 42 86 06 76

Stéphane Chapelle
29 Rue de Richelieu
75001 | +33 1 42 60 65 66

Sylvain Georges
4 Place des
Petits-Pères
75002 | +33 1 42 86 13 09

Odorantes
9 Rue Madame
75006 | +33 1 42 84 03 00

Adriane M
4 Rue Saint-Dominique
75007 | +33 1 42 22 22 46

Lachaume
103 Faubourg
Saint-Honoré
75008 | +33 1 42 60 59 74

Un peu, beaucoup...
18 Rue Pierre Guérin
75016 | +33 1 45 20 06 41

Furnishings
Declercq
15 Rue Étienne Marcel
75001 | +33 6 07 83 35 73

Thé & Beauté
Ladurée
232 Rue de Rivoli
75001 | +33 1 40 13 09 12

Christofle
18-20 Rue de la Paix
75002 | +33 1 42 65 62 43

L'Effet bulles
11 Passage Choiseul
75002 | +33 1 71 39 35 69

Merci
111 Boulevard
Beaumarchais
75003 | +33 1 42 77 00 33

Baccarat Maison
11 Place des États-Unis
75016 | +33 1 40 22 11 22

THE DINNER TABLE

*Clover Grill -
Jean-François Piège*
6 Rue Bailleul
75001 | +33 1 40 41 59 59

Les fines Gueules
43 Rue Croix-des-Petits-
Champs
75001 | +33 1 42 61 35 41

Senoble
11 Rue des
Petits-Champs
75001 | + 33 1 42 21 94 19

A. Noste
6bis Rue du
Quatre-Septembre
75002 | +33 1 47 03 91 91

Dépôt Légal
6 Rue des
Petits-Champs
75002 | +33 1 44 82 57 51

La Belle Époque
36 Rue des Petits-Champs
75002 | +33 1 42 96 33 33

*La Maison du
Croque-Monsieur*
108 Rue Réaumur
75002 | +33 1 42 36 97 76

Legrand filles & fils
1 Rue de la Banque
75002 | +33 1 42 60 07 12

Papa Boun Briocherie
21 Rue Marie Stuart
75002 | +33 1 42 60 14 40

Salatim
15 Rue des Jeûneurs
75002 | +33 1 42 36 30 03

Sushi-B Paris
5 Rue Rameau
75002 | +33 1 40 26 52 87

Grand Café Tortoni
45 Rue Saintonge
75003 | +33 1 42 72 28 92

Les Enfants Rouges
9, Rue de Beauce
75003 | +33 1 48 87 80 61

Vins des Pyrénées
25 Rue Beautreillis
75004 | +33 1 42 72 64 94

Les Bouquinistes
53 Quai des
Grands Augustins
75006 | +33 1 43 25 45 94

Cod House
1 Rue de Condé
75006 | +33 1 42 49 35 59

*Judy - La Cantine
qualitarienne*
18 Rue de Fleurus
75006 | +33 1 43 25 54 14

Le Comptoir du Relais
9 Carrefour de l'Odéon
75006 | +33 1 44 27 07 97

Café Constant
139 Rue Saint-Dominique
75007 | +33 1 47 53 73 34

Firmin le Barbier
20 Rue de Monttessuy
75007 | +33 1 45 51 21 55

Gaya by Pierre Gagnaire
44 Rue du Bac
75007 | +33 1 45 44 73 73

Bar des Théâtres
44 Rue Jean Goujon
75008 | +33 1 45 62 04 91

Caffè Artcurial
7 Rond-Point des
Champs-Élysées
Marcel-Dassault
75008 | +33 1 53 76 39 34

Chez Francis
7 Place de l'Alma
75008 | +33 1 47 20 86 83

*La Maison
du Danemark*
142 Avenue des
Champs-Élysées
75008 | +33 1 56 59 17 40

*The rooftop
of the Hôtel Marignan*
12 Rue Marignan
75008 | +33 1 40 76 34 56

Les Ambassadeurs
10 Place de la Concorde
75008 | +33 1 44 71 15 80

Mini Palais
3 Avenue
Winston Churchill
75008 | +33 1 42 56 42 42

Publicis Drugstore
133 Avenue des
Champs-Élysées
75008 | +33 1 44 43 77 64

*Crêperie
Les Cormorans*
63 Rue du Montparnasse
75014 | +33 1 43 35 26 68

La Terrasse - Hôtel Raphael
17 Avenue Kléber
75016 | +33 1 53 64 32 30

Monsieur Bleu
20 Avenue de New York
75016 | +33 1 47 20 90 47

*L'Huîtrade
of the Chiberta*
13 Rue Troyon
75017 | +33 1 44 09 95 85

Roca
31 Rue Guillaume Tell
75017 | +33 1 47 64 86 04

Bouillon Pigalle
22 Boulevard de Clichy
75018 | +33 1 42 59 69 31

Index

Acknowledgments

I'd like to thank the people who helped me create this book: Alessandra, Annabelle, Anne, Anne-Catherine, Annie, Aude, Barbara, Béatrice, Benedetta, Blanche, Brigitte, Carlo, Caroline, Catherine, Cécile, Chantal, Charles, Charlotte, Clara, Christian, Christophe, Daniela, Daniele, David, Denis, Donatella, Eduardo, Elena, Eliette, Elisha, Emilia, Fanny, François, Frédéric, Gabriela, Gabriele, Giacomo, Giovanni, Gisèle, Guylaine, Iryna, Isabelle, Jeanne, Jesse, Joëlle, Julien, Juliette, Karen, Kate, Laura, Lelia, Lou, Lucilla, Magalie, Marc, Maria Concetta, Maria Felice, Marion, Masha, Massimo, Maurizio, Maxime, Michael, Michel, Michela, Mireille, Myriam, Nick, Nicole, Nidia, Pamela, Paola, Pauline, Rebecca, Rita, Roberto, Rose, Rossella, Sandra, Samantha, Serena, Silvia, Silvio, Sophie, Stefano, Steve, Thierry, Valentina, Valeria, Valérie, Valerio, Vanessa, Virginia, Yves and all the people who were willing to answer my questions and be interviewed by me.

Special thanks to my husband, Bepi, who chose a Parisian to love; to my parents, who educated me and taught me the manners and inner elegance I'm proud of; to Giovanna, who gave me a mirror and Anna, who taught me to use it; to Maurizio, who has always supported me in my projects.

I would also like to thank all these beautiful brands and companies, all of them real French assets, for taking part in the realization of this work: Aigle, Baccarat, Barnes International, Bonton, Christofle, La Grande Épicerie de Paris, Lacoste, Ladurée, Le Bon Marché Rive Gauche, Paul, Petit Bateau, Pompadour, Repetto, Thé & Beauté by Ladurée, Yves Camdeborde.

My thanks also go to E. Marinella and Michela Bruni Reichlin, two great names of Italian luxury, for their presence in the volume.

Merci to Didier Villain, Frédéric Poletti, Irving Penn, Jennifer Sath, Laurent Parrault, Luxproductions, Matthieu de Martignac, Maxime de Pommereau, Taka Productions, Thierry Malty, Yves Duronsoy for kindly contributing their photographs.

This book wouldn't be so special without the help of Alessandra Ceriani, a gifted illustrator who has interpreted with elegance my Parisian woman's extravagant personality.

Many many thanks to the team of Mondadori Electa and Rizzoli New York for their professionalism and patience.

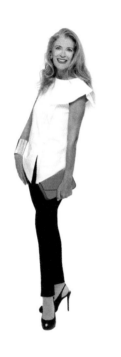

THE AUTHOR

After studying administration and management, Nathalie Peigney threw herself into the world of fashion and founded her own fashion house in Paris. As creator and manager, she traveled to the four corners of the globe to present her collections. Today she is a marketing consultant and journalist specializing in luxury products, men's fashion, and French gastronomy. Nathalie Peigney also edits the blog "Sophie the Parisian" (www.sophietheparisian.com), where she dialogues with a bunch of women and a man, critically presenting the Parisian way of life. She lives and works in Paris, Rome and the United States.

Illustrator
Alessandra Ceriani

Translations
SVP Traduction
Dov (Illinois)
Wee (Washington)
Michele (Arkansas)
Sylvia Notini (Italy)

Editorial Coordination
Valentina Lindon

Editor
Pamela Barr

Copy Editor
Valeria Perenze

Graphic Project and Cover
Anna Piccarreta - arachidepiu

Layout
Giorgia Dalla Pietà

Distributed in English throughout the World
by Rizzoli international Publications Inc.
300 Park Avenue South
New York, NY 10010, USA

ISBN: 978-8-89-181792-1

www.sophietheparisian.com
www.facebook.com/sophietheparisian
www.instagram.com/sophietheparisian
www.pinterest.com.au/SophieParisian

Libri Illustrati Rizzoli
© 2018 Mondadori Electa S.p.A., Milano
All rights reserved
First edition: October 2018

ISO 9001
Mondadori Electa S.p.A. is certified for the Quality
Management System by Bureau Veritas Italia S.p.A.,
in compliance with UNI EN ISO 9001.

This book respects the environment
The paper used was produced using wood from forests managed
to strict environmental standards; the companies involved
guarantee sustainable production certified environmentally.

Printed in May 2018 by Errestampa, Italy.

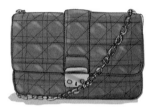